10-MINUTE PILATES

The ultimate way to a better body

Health&Fitness MAGAZINE

Words Caroline Sandry
Photography Henry Carter, Thinkstock
Clothing from a selection at Wellicious (wellicious.com),
USA Pro (store.usapro.co.uk), Lululemon (lululemon.co.uk),
Striders Edge (stridersedge.com)
Hair & make up Julia Wade @ Artistic Licence

Editor Mary Comber
Art Editor Lucy Pinto
Chief Sub-Editor Sheila Reid
Digital Production Manager Nicky Baker

MagBook Publisher Dharmesh Mistry
Operations Director Robin Ryan
MagBook Advertising Manager Simone Daws
Managing Director of Advertising Julian Lloyd-Evans
Newstrade Director David Barker
Managing Director of Enterprise Martin Belson
Publisher Nicola Bates
Group Publisher Russell Blackman
Group Managing Director Ian Westwood
Chief Operating Officer Brett Reynolds
Group Finance Director Ian Leggett
Chief Executive James Tye
Chairman Felix Dennis

MAGBOOK

10-MINUTE PILATES ISBN1-78106-290-0
To license this product, please contact Carlotta Serantoni on +44 (0) 20 79076550 or email carlotta_serantoni@dennis.co.uk
To syndicate content from this product, please contact Anj Dosaj Halai on +44(0) 20 7907 6132
or email anj_dosaj-halai@dennis. co.uk

While every care was taken during the production of this MagBook, the publishers cannot be held responsible for the accuracy of the information or any consequence arising from it. Dennis Publishing takes no responsibility for the companies advertising in this MagBook. The paper used within this MagBook is produced from sustainable fibre, manufactured by mills with a valid chain of custody. Printed in China.

The health and diet information presented in this book is an educational resource and is not intended as a substitute for medical advice.

KNOW IT

The sense of wellbeing that can be achieved through physical and mental self awareness along with a more relaxed mind and soul is a powerful feeling.

NEXGEN® SPORTS MULTIVITAMIN

Nexgen® Sports Multivitamin has been formulated for those undertaking regular training or exercise with the highest quality chelated minerals for superior absorption. This spectrum of ingredients contributes to normal muscle function, a reduction of tiredness and fatigue, normal energy-yielding metabolism, normal protein synthesis, normal function of the immune system and the maintenance of normal bones. It also contributes to normal absorption of calcium and phosphorous as well as normal blood calcium levels.

A TOTAL OF 28 KEY INGREDIENTS

Do you know of another brand that includes all of the following ingredients? Magnesium, natural vitamin K2-MK7, vitamin D3 and a range of micronutrients including DeltaGold® delta-tocotrienols, Lyc-O-Mato® (natural lycopene), BIOLUT™ lutein esters, grapeseed extract, green tea extract, Selenium SeLECT® and natural coenzyme Q10.

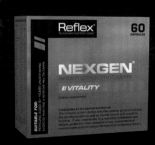

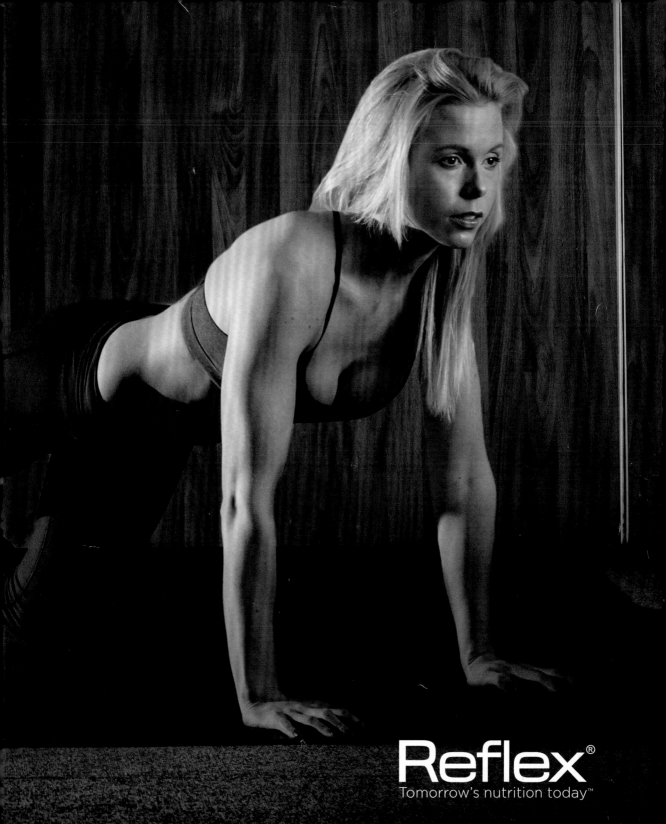

Reflex®
Tomorrow's nutrition today™

Contents

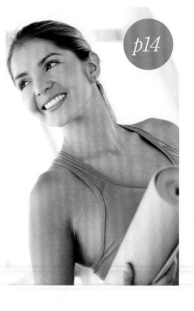

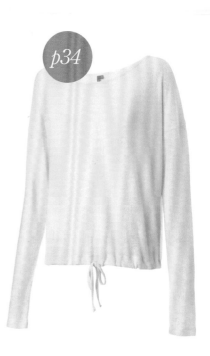

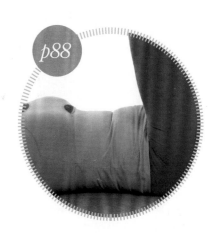

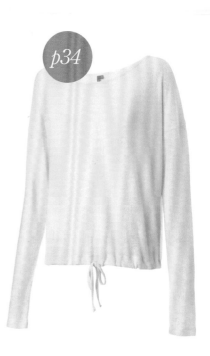

p34

p58

p88

Hello...

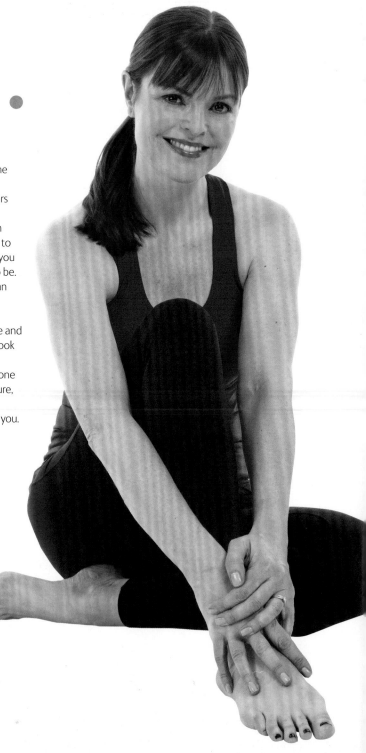

Welcome to *10-Minute Pilates* and the start of a better body. I've been teaching Pilates for the past 12 years and have witnessed the amazing changes and transformations it can bring. Pilates is a unique system of exercise that allows you to identify and address any imbalances in your body, helping you to get back to the real you, the way nature intended you to be. Practising Pilates regularly will give you an enviable long, lean look and help you to stay strong and flexible for life.

10-Minute Pilates is the ideal solution for today's time-pressed woman, who's busy juggling career, family, exercise and home life. The super-effective exercises you'll find in this book are designed to give you maximum results in the minimum time, so you won't waste a second! Whether you want to tone up all over, target your trouble zones or improve your posture, there's a solution for you.

Let's turn the page and get started on the road to a better you.

ABOUT CAROLINE

Caroline Sandry is a qualified personal trainer, Pilates and yoga teacher with over 12 years' experience. Her passion for exercise and wellbeing has seen her present 13 Pilates and fitness DVDs as well as writing two other fitness titles.

Always striving to increase her knowledge, Caroline has studied with experts all over the world. 'I am in awe of the human body, it's truly amazing. I hope that by passing on my knowledge and passion I can motivate others to improve their health and their lives,' she says.

Caroline has a one-year-old daughter and also specialises in pre- and post-natal Pilates. For more info about Caroline, go to www.carolinesandry.com or read her blog *All things healthy* at www.carolinesandry.wordpress.com.

Your Pilates holiday
Introducing the Azul Experience...

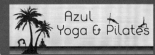
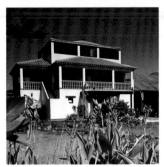
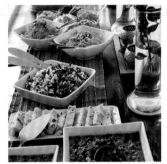
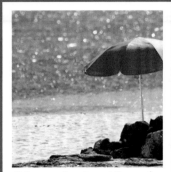
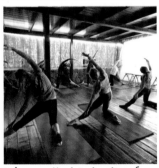
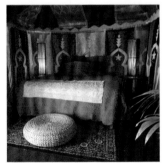
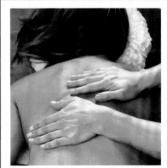
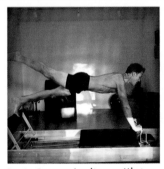
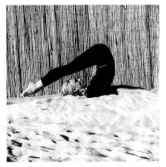
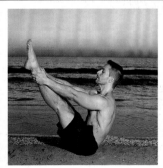

How to use this book

This guide offers everything you need to practise Pilates at home, from step-by-step instruction to 10-minute workouts. Ready to go? Read these guidelines first to get the most from your practice

We all lead busy lives which is why I've created *10-minute Pilates* to help you shape up quickly, easily and safely. To get the full benefits, it's essential you learn the basics and build up your from there. *10-minute Pilates* sets out the principles of Pilates with step-by-step photographs and instructions.

Take time to read through the book first, getting to know the principles and details of the practice.

Once you've got the foundations in place and are familiar with the exercises, you can add the workouts into your daily life. Alternatively, dip in and out at your own pace or build your own tailored workouts.

Always do a warm-up before each session, to prepare your body for the workout and help prevent injury. End each session with a cool down and stretch, to relax your body and help it recover for the next session.

Discover Pilates

Learn about the history of Pilates and why it's hailed as the ultimate exercise system. Discover the benefits it has to offer your body and mind, and how it can fit into your busy daily life.

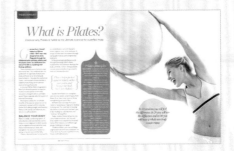

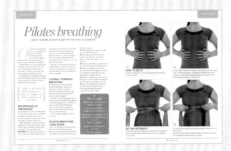

Learn the basics

Here you'll learn the essential breathing and postural techniques that make Pilates effective. You'll also learn several key moves that create the foundations of all other Pilates moves.

Perfect the moves

I'll walk you through each move, step-by-step, with clear photos and instructions. You'll also find modifications for your experience and ability, plus teaching tips to help perfect your alignment.

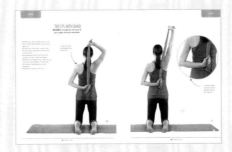

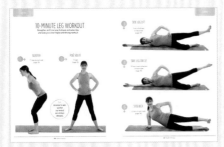

Try the workouts

You've got the basics, now you can start practising my 10-minute Pilates workouts. Choose them to suit your goals – from sculpting your arms to toning your tummy – or mix and match.

Pilates directory

This is your one-stop directory for all things Pilates, including finding a qualified teacher, favourite kit, clothes and websites. Start today and look forward to a fit, toned new you!

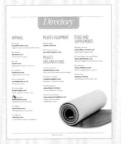

What is Pilates?

Discover why Pilates is hailed as the ultimate exercise for a perfect body

German-born Joseph Hubertus Pilates (1883-1967) was way ahead of his time. Plagued through his childhood with asthma, rickets and rheumatic fever, he dedicated the rest of his life to studying and finding wellness.

Pilates studied human anatomy, yoga and martial arts. This, combined with his professions as a gymnast, body builder, diver and boxer led to his total body transformation – he posed for anatomical charts – and a system of exercise that is hailed by many today as the ultimate exercise for a perfect body.

In the mid 1920s, Pilates emigrated to New York where he opened an exercise studio and soon gained an enviable reputation among the dance and ballet world. Pilates originally called his system of exercise Contrology.

Word spread about the remarkable benefits of his exercise system and it has continued to spread until this very day. Known for building strength and flexibility, Pilates is still used by top ballerinas and dancers as well as athletes.

BALANCE YOUR BODY

Pilates is a body conditioning system of precisely executed exercises that set the body in correct alignment so that muscles can be targeted and exercised effectively. Pilates improves posture, tones and strengthens the body and is known for giving a long, lean look and flat belly.

Pilates is also well known for its benefits as a rehabilitation tool and helping to protect against injury, aches and pains. It brings the body back into balance through easing tight muscles and strengthening weak ones.

In his pioneering book *Return to Life through Contrology* (1945), Pilates explained that his technique 'develops the body uniformly, corrects wrong postures, restores physical vitality, invigorates the mind and elevates the spirit'.

> *Pilates helps protect against injury, aches and pains and brings the body back into balance*

Studies show Pilates can strengthen your immune system, protecting you from illness. It can even boost your sex life by strengthening your pelvic floor.

All Pilates exercises begin from your centre or 'powerhouse', helping to develop a strong core. This 'centring' or focusing also helps to connect your mind with your body, shutting out external stress and creating a calming effect.

Today, modern Pilates still teaches the same fundamental exercises but, with time, experts have adapted and modified some of the moves to suit different age groups, body types and goals.

10-Minute Pilates uses many of Pilates' original exercises with some variations I've drawn from my 15 years' experience in the fitness and health industry.

Pilates principles

ALIGNMENT: If one part of the body is misaligned, it affects the whole body. Working in correct alignment helps improve the body's function and wellbeing.

BREATHING: Pilates exercises are co-ordinated with the breath to aid control. Breathing is full and relaxed to help power the body.

CONCENTRATION: Focusing the mind and fully committing to each move helps ensure maximum benefits and encourages relaxation.

CONTROL: Every Pilates move is executed with careful control. Knowing what each part of the body is doing allows you to exercise more effectively. The slower the move, the harder you have to work.

FLOW: Using slow, controlled, flowing movements synchronised with the breath enables the body to move as nature intended.

CENTRING: All Pilates moves begin from the centre or core. Pilates called it the 'girdle of strength' or 'powerhouse'. Performing Pilates exercises helps develop an internal corset, supporting your spine and flattening your abs.

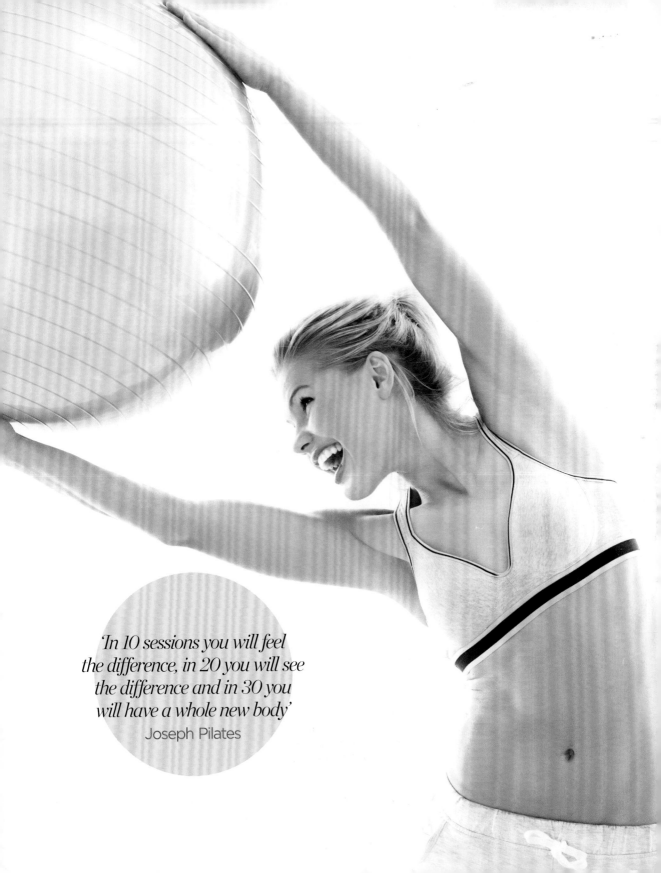

'In 10 sessions you will feel
the difference, in 20 you will see
the difference and in 30 you
will have a whole new body'
Joseph Pilates

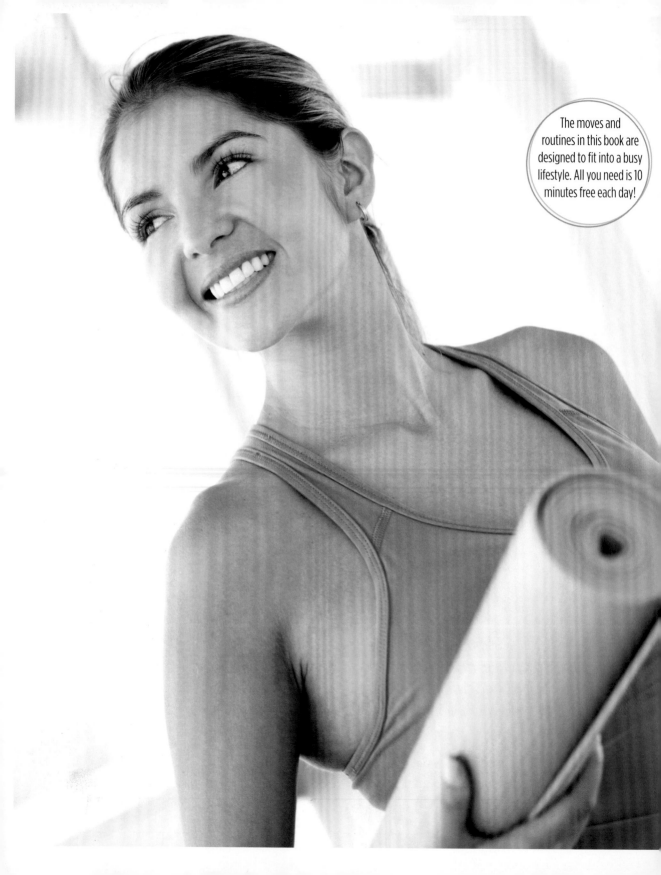

The moves and routines in this book are designed to fit into a busy lifestyle. All you need is 10 minutes free each day!

Pilates for modern life

Here's how Pilates can help you shape up – however busy you are

Modern life is not kind to the human body. Machines have taken over many of the chores that previous generations cursed, such as scrubbing floors and clothes, walking or cycling to work in the rain and snow and fetching and carrying wood and water. While it's wonderful that we don't have to endure these hardships, the cost to our bodies has been huge and our posture, weight, health and wellbeing have suffered enormously as a result.

Sitting at computers, desks and cars has given us hunched backs, round shoulders and fat stomachs. Slumping on the sofa watching TV has given us weak backs, flabby bottoms and poor circulation. These factors lead to back and neck pain, headaches and increased stress caused by poor breathing. Slump over and try to take a nice deep breath. Now stand up tall and try again. Can you feel the difference?

GOOD FOR POSTURE

Pilates can help to address many modern ailments and is routinely prescribed by physiotherapists, doctors and osteopaths as a remedy for back, shoulder, postural and joint problems. The precise, controlled nature of Pilates makes the exercises extremely safe for everyone and the focus on body and joint alignment can help undo postural problems.

Many issues that people take to their GP, including back and neck pain and urinary incontinence, can be rectified with regular Pilates exercises. It strengthens where the body is weak and lengthens where it is tight.

Developing core strength helps prevent back pain and enables the body to move more freely. Pilates also ensures the spine is regularly moved safely through all of its

> { *The precise, controlled nature of Pilates makes the exercises extremely safe for everyone* }

natural range of motion – flexion, extension and rotation help it stay supple and strong.

Pilates is also frequently hailed by many a celebrity as their exercise of choice for a slim but strong 'red-carpet-ready' body. It's perfect for toning trouble zones such as bottom, thighs, arms and tummy.

10 Minute Pilates is written with our busy modern lives in mind – in spite of our time-saving machines, we've probably never been more time deprived! The moves and routines in this book are designed to fit into your lifestyle no matter how full your day. All you need is a little space – and 10 minutes of course!

TAKE 10 MINUTES

Almost everyone can find 10 minutes in a day, and those precious moments will help you to stay young, strong and supple. Use the upper body moves (page 52) during your lunch break to help prevent hunched, tight shoulders. Try the Total Body workout (page 112) first thing in the morning to energise you to set you up for the day. The core exercises (page 82) and stretches (page 112) will help ease out postural 'kinks' from the day and calm your mind for sleep.

The moves in this book can be performed anywhere – in your office at lunchtime or beside your bed at night. What matters most is that you actually DO the exercises to help you get the most out of your busy life and keep your body and mind young and flexible!

Benefits of Pilates

- ◆ Tightens and tones your body
- ◆ Calms your mind
- ◆ Strengthens your spine
- ◆ Improves flexibility
- ◆ Creates a long, lean look
- ◆ Improves co-ordination
- ◆ Flattens your belly
- ◆ Improves your posture
- ◆ Corrects imbalances
- ◆ Prevents injury
- ◆ Improves athletic performance
- ◆ Heightens mind-body awareness

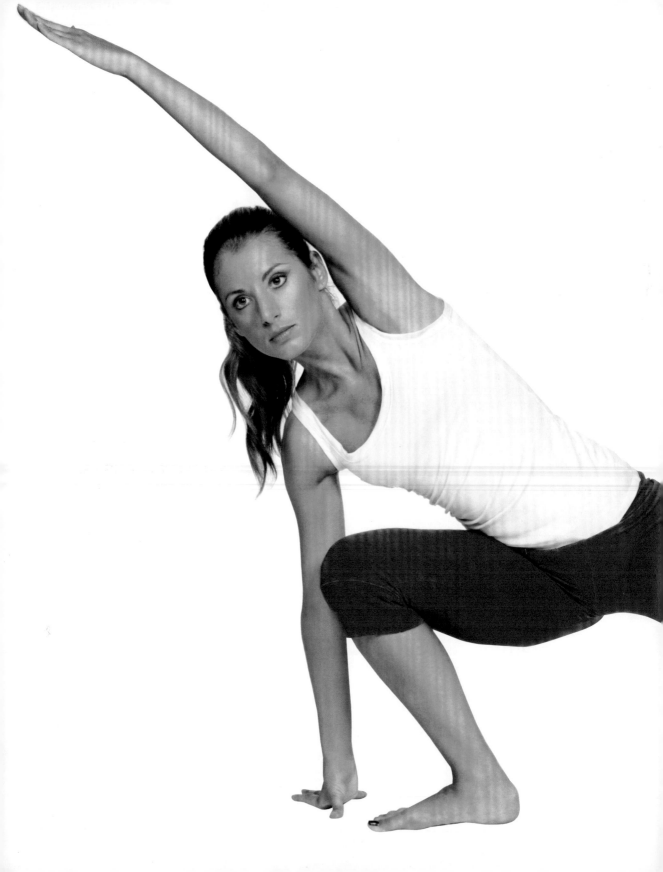

THE FOUNDATIONS

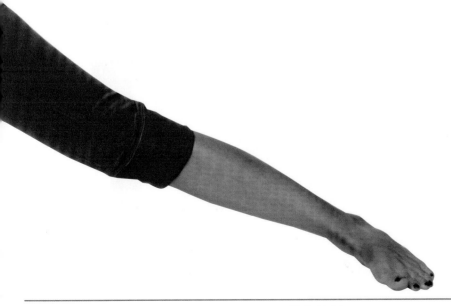 The following pages are the most important in this book. You'll learn the fundamental foundations of Pilates on which you'll build your practice.

Over the course of these pages, you'll learn the correct posture, breathing and alignment you need to practise Pilates. You'll also learn about your core and why it's key to good health. It's said that the best things in life come to those who wait and this is true with Pilates!

In my experience, the Pilates breath can take more than a few sessions before it starts to feel natural as most of us have forgotten how to breathe properly. You might find you're holding your breath when you're doing the exercises. If so, just relax, follow the instructions and remember that practice makes perfect!

Pilates posture

Discover the secret of perfect poise and
how Pilates can help you achieve it

As you read this page, take a minute to check your posture. Are you sitting up straight or slumped on the sofa or over a desk? For most of us, good posture is tiring to maintain for more than a few minutes. Our modern day lifestyle has weakened our postural muscles and put our bodies out of alignment. Poor posture not only leads to fatigue and backache, it makes you appear shorter and rounder too.

Try standing tall with your shoulders open, your abdominals pulled slightly in and breathe more deeply. You'll instantly notice that you look taller with a flatter stomach. You'll also feel more alert and energised. Ideally this is how we should all carry ourselves – and this is what Pilates can help you achieve.

Pilates has a great reputation for improving posture and rightly so! The exercises in this book will help to open your shoulders and flatten your abs. They will strengthen weak postural muscles, particularly around your mid-section and upper back, and stretch tight, shortened muscles, particularly in the front of your chest and your lower back.

Practise Pilates regularly and you'll notice that you start to sit naturally and stand taller without any effort. Pilates can give you the natural poise and elegance of a dancer. But first you need to learn the basics..

HOW TO FIND PERFECT POISE

Stand sideways on to a mirror and be honest with yourself! Try to adopt your usual posture, then compare it with the photo on the opposite page (far right). Don't try to adopt a very different posture immediately as this will feel unnatural and may strain certain muscles. Just identify your weaknesses, such as round shoulders or pot belly, and feel grateful that you're about to improve them!

A quick fix for all posture types is to imagine that you have a string coming from the top of your head, and that an invisible force is pulling that string up. Try this now. Stand in your usual posture, sideways to a mirror. Now draw your whole body upwards imagining that string, then check the mirror again. It's simple but effective!

▶ In this photo we can see that the lower back is very arched, making the stomach round forward and the bottom stick out. This type of poor posture puts a strain on the lumbar spine and affects the balance of the whole body.

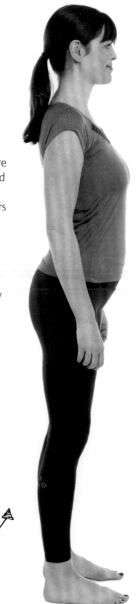

X

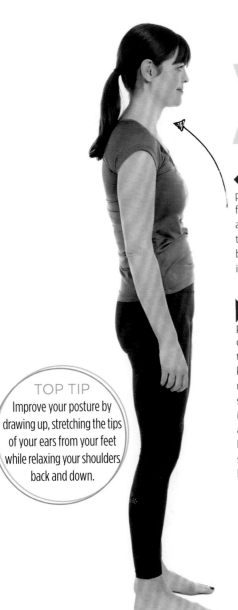

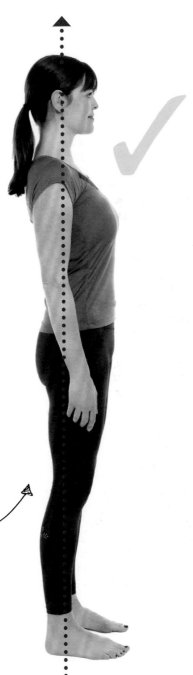

◀ Here we see the 'sofa slump' posture with rounded shoulders, a flattened bottom, weak, rounded abs and head tilting forwards. This type of posture strains the upper back and neck and doesn't improve with age!

▶ This is close to the ideal posture. You can see that the line drawn through the body passes through the ear, shoulder, hip, knee and ankle. The spine maintains its ideal neutral 'S' shaped curves and the eye line is straight ahead. With this alignment, the abs are more likely to work effectively, supporting the spine, and the body is more balanced.

TOP TIP
Improve your posture by drawing up, stretching the tips of your ears from your feet while relaxing your shoulders back and down.

Pilates breathing

Learn to breathe properly to get the most from your practice

One of the key principles of Pilates is the breath. In an ideal world, we'd all breath fully into our abdomen with relaxed shoulders. Watch a baby breathe for a lesson in how we should do it properly!

Unfortunately stress, poor posture and bad habits mean that, more often than not, we take shallow breaths into our upper chest, tensing our shoulders and increasing general feelings of stress.

Controlling and maximising your breath will not only help you perform your Pilates moves more fully, it will also boost your wellbeing and aid relaxation.

Exhale on the effort as this helps your deep core muscles to activate and power each move

IMPORTANCE OF THE EXHALE

In basic Pilates, we use the exhale breath for most of our movements – remember to **E**xhale on the **E**xertion or **E**ffort –because this helps our deep core muscles to activate and power each move.

When exhaling, your body is trying to squeeze out the air, reducing the volume of the lungs and thereby the size of the 'container' – your ribs and tummy.
TRY THIS: Stand up, place your hands on your stomach and take a deep breath in,

relaxing your abs. Now blow out through pursed lips and keep blowing out ALL the air. You should feel your deep abs tighten and draw in as they try to expel the air. The same thing happens when you cough. Your abs contract to force the air out of your lungs.

We want to use this natural 'flattening' or 'tightening' of the abs as we exercise because this will protect and support our spine and help to build a natural girdle or corset of strength.

LATERAL THORACIC BREATHING

For Pilates exercises, we use lateral thoracic breathing or sideways rib breathing. This means taking your breath into the sides of your rib cage, keeping your shoulders relaxed and your core gently engaged.

This type of breathing enables you to perform the exercises while keeping your core gently engaged. If you inhale into your stomach while performing an exercise, your tummy muscles will expand, meaning that you'll lose your navel to spine contraction.

See the diagrams opposite on how to do this.

PILATES BREATHING LYING DOWN

Here's how to employ the Pilates breath when you're doing floor exercises.
● Lie on your back with your knees bent, feet and knees hip-width apart

and your shoulders relaxed.
● Take a deep breath in and then 'sigh' out to release any tension.
● Allow your body to melt into the mat. Try to relax your rib cage and sacrum – back of your pelvis – on to the mat.
● Relax your shoulders and neck and feel that your collar bones are wide and flat.
● Inhale and imagine your rib cage expanding without allowing your back to arch or your ribs to lift off the mat, and keeping your shoulders relaxed.
● Breathe in through your nose and out through your mouth. Slightly pursing your lips can help you to engage your core.
● Take several breaths in this way and, when you are comfortable, try the breathing while keeping a gentle contraction of navel to spine.

The benefits
● Helps to relax your muscles and ease tension

● Encourages effective oxygenation of the blood.

● Encourages the engagement of the deep transversus abdominis muscle

● Improves posture

● Supports good movement patterns

● Focuses the mind

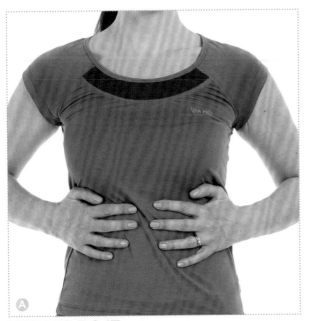

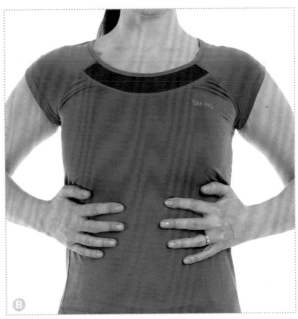

HOW TO DO IT

◆ Place your hands on to your rib cage with your fingertips just touching (A).

◆ Take a deep breath in and feel your ribs expand out to the side – like an umbrella opening – pushing your fingertips apart (B).

◆ Repeat several breaths while keeping your shoulders relaxed and navel gently drawn in to your spine.

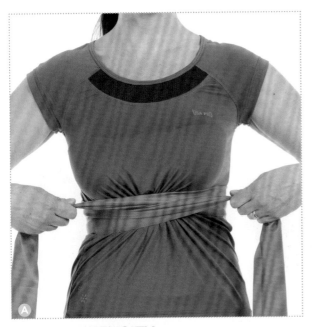

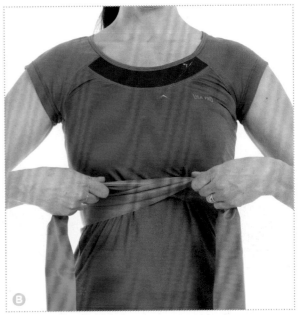

UP THE INTENSITY

◆ Now increase the intensity by wrapping a flex band tightly around your ribs. Cross the ends over each other and hold as shown (A).

◆ Inhale and expand your ribs sideways against the resistance of the band (B).

◆ Repeat several breaths while keeping your shoulders relaxed and navel gently drawn towards your spine.

Finding neutral

Before beginning your exercises, put your spine into a neutral position

In Pilates we talk about a neutral spine. But what does neutral really mean? Your spine is made up of 24 articulating vertebrae which should form a nice gentle 'S' shape rather than the '?' shape of a hunched upper back and flat lower back that we see so often these days.

This 'S' shape is your spine's neutral position and, when in correct alignment, it provides natural shock absorption from impact, allowing the weight of your body to be transferred through the centre of each joint. However, if your body is out of alignment, its weight will be displaced, and therefore put a strain on your vertebrae and joints.

A neutral spine and pelvis enables your limbs to move freely and naturally. If, for example your pelvis is tilted forwards – creating a large arch in the lower back – this can affect the muscles of your back, bottom and thighs and can lead to weakness, tightness and even injury.

Ideally, we would all have a neutral posture but modern life gets in the way. However, by doing Pilates you are off to a very good start. And as your posture and alignment starts to improve, you'll notice it's easier to maintain a neutral spine as you go about your daily business.

Many Pilates exercises are performed in neutral. However, some moves require you to imprint your spine on the floor instead – flattening your back rather than being in neutral – to create a safer position for challenging your abs.

FIND A NEUTRAL SPINE LYING DOWN

1 Lie with your knees bent and feet hip-width apart. Press your lower back flat on the floor.

2 Arch your lower back off the floor. Continue four or five times making the movements smaller and smaller.

3 Finally, settle at a point where your back is neither flat on the floor nor arched off the floor but in between.

Once in neutral, you can feel with your hands that your pubic bone and your hip bones are more or less level. Remember that no two bodies are the same, and the arch under your back might look bigger if you have a larger bottom.

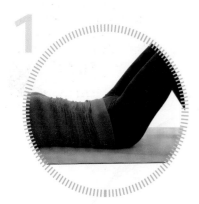

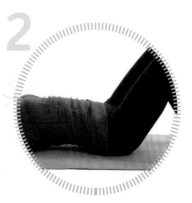

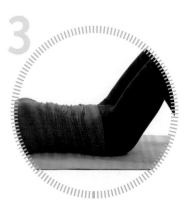

TOP TIP: Imagine you have a big bowl of soup on your stomach. You don't want the soup to tip out of the front or back of the bowl but to lie flat.

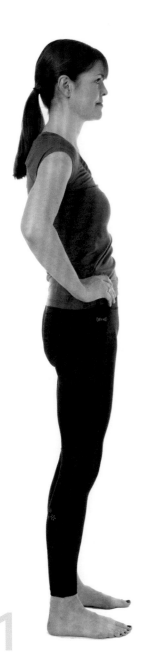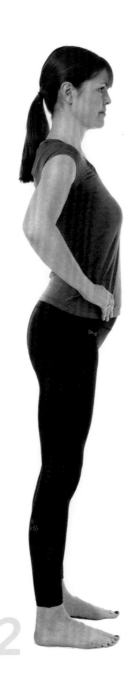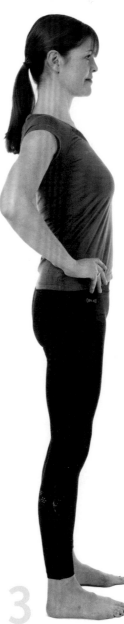

FIND NEUTRAL IN STANDING

Try this side on to a mirror:
Stand with your feet hip-width apart and your knees soft

1 First tuck your tailbone under, flattening out your lower back.

2 Now arch your back by sticking your bottom out. Move four to five times in each direction making the movements smaller and smaller until you come to rest in the middle.

3 At this point your back should have a gentle curve, and if you place your hands on your pelvis you will feel that your pubic bone is in line with your hips bones. Watch what happens to your stomach. If you arch your back too much your stomach will poke out making you look much bigger!

Note that your shoulders should also be in a neutral position, with the shoulder blades drawn slightly towards each other and down. You can imagine that you are sliding your shoulder blades down towards a single back pocket in the middle of your jeans.

1   2   3

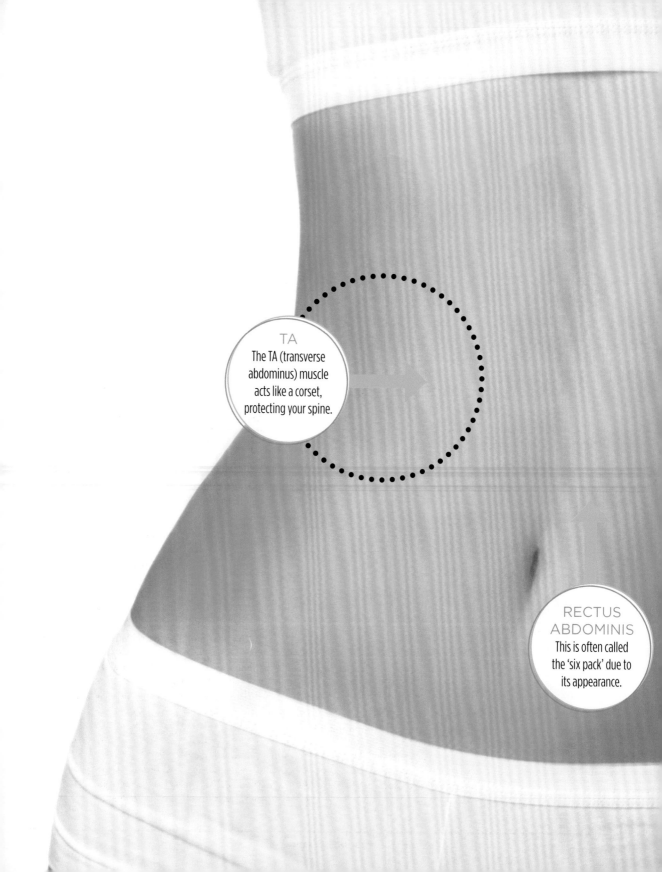

TA
The TA (transverse abdominus) muscle acts like a corset, protecting your spine.

RECTUS ABDOMINIS
This is often called the 'six pack' due to its appearance.

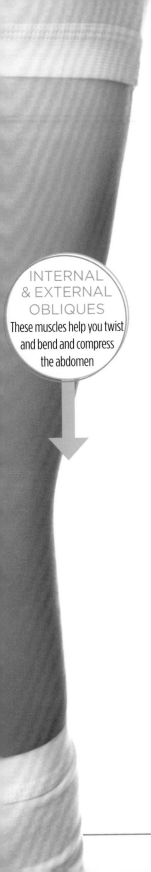

About your core

Discover the secret to a flat tummy and inner strength

INTERNAL & EXTERNAL OBLIQUES
These muscles help you twist and bend and compress the abdomen

Your core is the centre of your body and comprises all the muscles in and around your trunk. Having a strong core is key to a healthy, functional body. What good would a crane be if its central body was weak? It would bend under the smallest weight, and this analogy can be applied to your spine.

The stronger your core is, the more weight you can lift with your arms, the more power you can push through your legs and the safer and more stable your spine and pelvis will be.

All Pilates movements begin at the core. By connecting to your deep core muscles when exercising, your pelvis and spine will be supported, helping to prevent injury and poor movement patterns. Strengthening your core with Pilates will tone all the layers of muscles around your mid section, drawing in your waist, flattening your tummy and strengthening your pelvic floor.

HOW TO CONNECT

We're all familiar with the rectus abdominis muscle, commonly known as the six pack muscle due to its appearance. This is the most superficial ab muscle and consists of two vertical bands of muscle which flex your spine, bringing your chest towards your hips and vice versa.

Beneath this lies the oblique muscles – internal and external obliques – which run diagonally and allow your spine to side bend and twist as well as stabilising the trunk.

Deeper still lies the transversus abdominis (TA) which is like a corset that wraps around your waist. This muscle draws your navel in towards your spine. The TA does not move your spine but supports it.

The TA works in harmony with another set of deep core muscles, collectively known as the pelvic floor. These muscles are shaped like a sling, and offer support for your pelvis and internal organs. You might have already discovered these muscles if you've ever tried to stop yourself from going to the loo or if you've had a baby and have practised your post-natal pelvic floor exercises.

ZIP IT UP

Throughout this book, you'll be reminded to 'draw navel to spine' and this action should feel as if you're gently drawing your pelvic floor upwards – internally – and your tummy button inwards as if you're zipping up a very tight pair of jeans. This action will not cause your body to move, but will flatten your tummy and stabilise your spine and pelvis.

Practise now by placing your hands on your stomach, taking a deep breath in and then exhaling slowly and fully, drawing your tummy button in as you exhale.

Each Pilates exercise should begin from your core, and you'll be instructed to 'inhale to prepare' (body and mind) 'exhale and engage navel to spine' as you flow into your exercise. Don't worry if it feels unnatural to begin with – practice makes perfect!

BASIC MOVES

The following Pilates exercises lay the foundations for many of the moves in this book. It's important to be familiar with them first. They will take your spine through flexion, extension and rotation; mobilise your shoulders; open your chest and strengthen your core. Regular practice of these exercises will help keep your body in balance for many years to come.

SCISSOR ARMS

Benefits: mobilises your shoulder joints and improves your posture

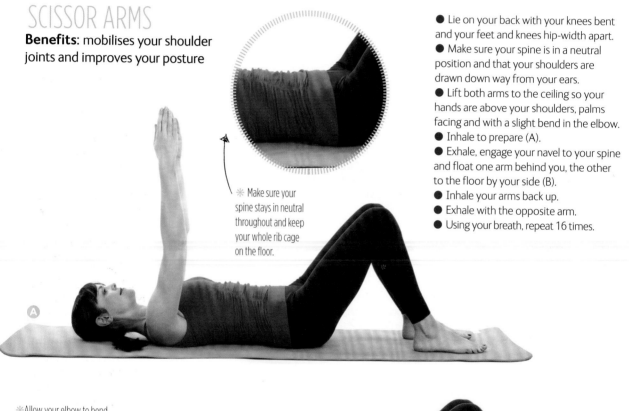

✳ Make sure your spine stays in neutral throughout and keep your whole rib cage on the floor.

● Lie on your back with your knees bent and your feet and knees hip-width apart.
● Make sure your spine is in a neutral position and that your shoulders are drawn down way from your ears.
● Lift both arms to the ceiling so your hands are above your shoulders, palms facing and with a slight bend in the elbow.
● Inhale to prepare (A).
● Exhale, engage your navel to your spine and float one arm behind you, the other to the floor by your side (B).
● Inhale your arms back up.
● Exhale with the opposite arm.
● Using your breath, repeat 16 times.

✳Allow your elbow to bend softly to help your shoulder relax as you move. Keep the movement soft and flowing.

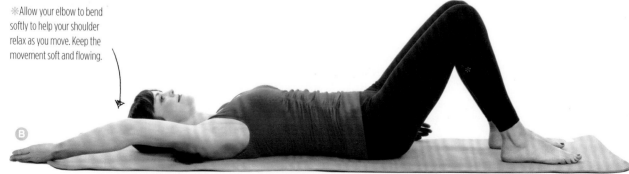

SPINAL TWIST

Benefits: mobilises your spine, particularly your thoracic spine (upper back), improves your posture and stretches your shoulders and chest

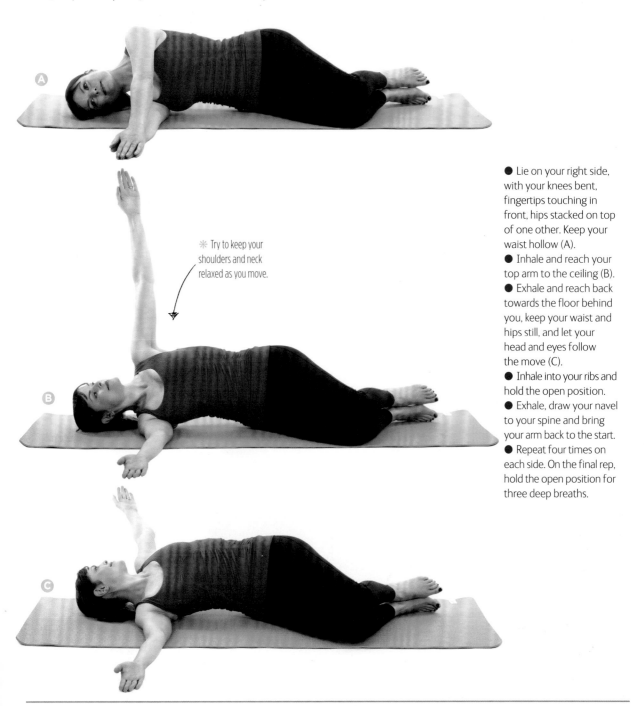

✳ Try to keep your shoulders and neck relaxed as you move.

● Lie on your right side, with your knees bent, fingertips touching in front, hips stacked on top of one other. Keep your waist hollow (A).

● Inhale and reach your top arm to the ceiling (B).

● Exhale and reach back towards the floor behind you, keep your waist and hips still, and let your head and eyes follow the move (C).

● Inhale into your ribs and hold the open position.

● Exhale, draw your navel to your spine and bring your arm back to the start.

● Repeat four times on each side. On the final rep, hold the open position for three deep breaths.

PELVIC TILT

Benefits: mobilises your lumbar spine, flattens your
abs and strengthens your pelvic floor and core

● Lie on your back with your knees bent
with your feet and knees hip-width apart
and spine in neutral. Inhale to prepare (A).
● Exhale and draw your pelvic floor up
and your navel in as you tuck your tailbone
under. At the same time press your lower
back into the floor (B).
● Inhale and lengthen back into a
neutral position.
● Continue for 10 to 15 breaths.

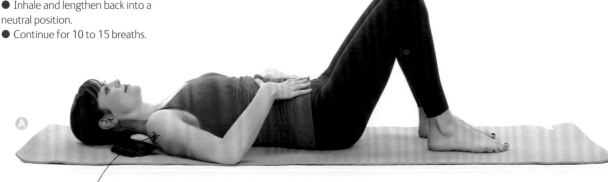

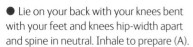

✳ Try to keep your
shoulders and neck
relaxed as you move.

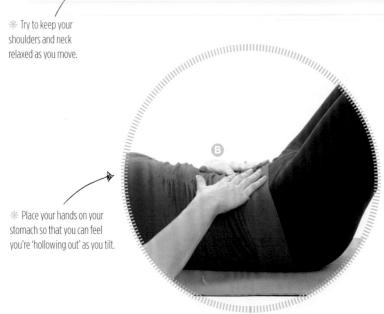

✳ Place your hands on your
stomach so that you can feel
you're 'hollowing out' as you tilt.

BASIC AB CURL

Benefits: strengthens your core and flattens your abs

✳ Try to keep your pelvis very still and your thighs and pelvis relaxed or your legs might try to 'help you' by taking the emphasis off your abs.

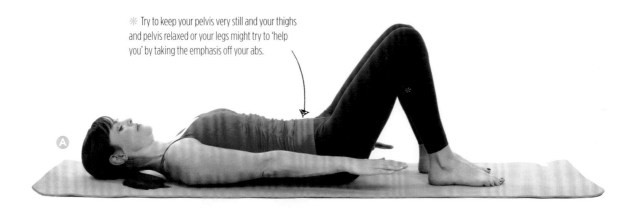

Ⓐ

✳ If you feel your neck is straining, place one hand behind your head to gently support its weight.

✳ Think of bringing your rib cage towards your hip bones as you lift.

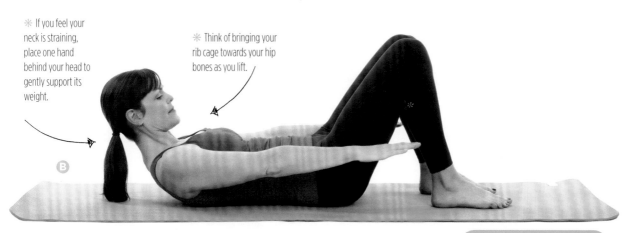

Ⓑ

● Lie on your back with your knees bent and feet and knees hip-width apart.
● Begin in neutral spine with your shoulders drawn away from your ears.
● Inhale and gently lengthen the back of your neck, tucking your chin slightly (A).
● Exhale, engage your navel to your spine and draw your shoulder blades down as you contract your abs to fold your head and shoulders off the mat while reaching your fingers down to your toes. Keep your arms off the mat (B).
● Inhale and maintain your navel to spine connection as you take a shallow breath into the sides of your ribs.
● Exhale and return your head, shoulders and arms to the mat.
● Using your breath, do eight reps.
● To progress, on the final repetition, stay in the 'up' position and add 12 crunches, exhaling each time you lift a little higher off the floor.

VARIATIONS
1. Place a pillow or ball between your knees and squeeze as you curl up.
2. Place both hands behind your head.
3. Place both hands in front of your head with your fingertips touching your forehead.
4. In the 'up' position, lift both arms up so your upper arms are beside your ears, maintaining the ab crunch. This is an advanced move.

TABLE TOP LEGS

Benefits: stabilises your pelvis and spine and strengthens your core

● Lie on your back with your knees bent and feet and knees hip-width apart with your spine and pelvis in neutral.

● Exhale and engage your navel to your spine, keeping your hips still as you lift one leg so your knee is above your hip and bent to 90° – like the leg and top of a table (A).

● Inhale and keep a stable spine and pelvis as you lower your foot to the lift-off spot.

● Repeat on the other side and continue alternating your legs for 12 reps.

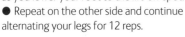

※ This exercise might seem very simple, but the challenge is to keep a neutral spine and flat tummy throughout while preventing your hips from rolling from side to side.

TO PROGRESS

● To progress, do as above, but lift one leg and then the other one on exhale. Inhale to hold in a table top then exhale to lower one leg then the other on a second exhale. Keep your spine very still as you lift and lower your second leg.

BASIC BREAST STROKE

Benefits: mobilises your spine, particularly your thoracic spine or upper back, and strengthens your postural muscles around your shoulder girdle

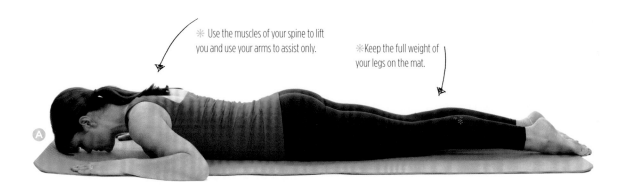

✳ Use the muscles of your spine to lift you and use your arms to assist only.

✳ Keep the full weight of your legs on the mat.

A

● Lie on your stomach with your legs drawn together and your arms bent on the floor – finger tips approximately in line with your nose (A).
● Inhale to prepare.
● Exhale and gently draw your navel to your spine as you push your hands into the floor and draw your shoulder blades down, away from your

ears. At the same time extend your head and shoulders off the floor while keeping your bottom rib in contact with the floor (B).
● Inhale to hold up and try to lengthen the front of your chest away from your toes.
● Exhale to lower yourself back to the start.
● Repeat eight times.

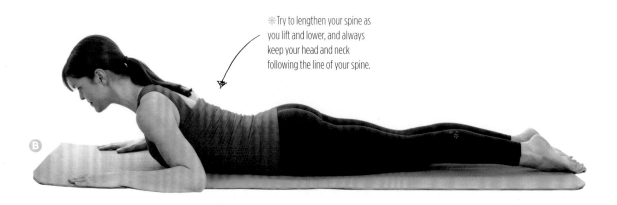

✳ Try to lengthen your spine as you lift and lower, and always keep your head and neck following the line of your spine.

B

THE WORKOUTS

✳ Now you've learned the basics, you're ready for a daily workout. In this section you'll find the moves to tone up all over and improve your wellbeing. This book is divided into sections to target your trouble zones: bum, arms, legs, abs, back and total body. I've created six 10-minute workouts – one for each zone. Need to tone up your tummy? Have a look at the Ab Workout (page 82). Stiff back and poor posture? Try the Back Workout (page 96). Need to tone your whole body? Try the Total Body Workout (page 112).

For those days when you're 'in the zone', do a few workouts together. Begin with the warm up then try the Arms, followed by the Legs and Abs moves for a 30-minute session. These gentle exercises can be performed every day. My only advice is to listen to your body! Remember the principles of Pilates (page 12) and if you can't complete an exercise with great form or you're losing concentration and flow – stop!

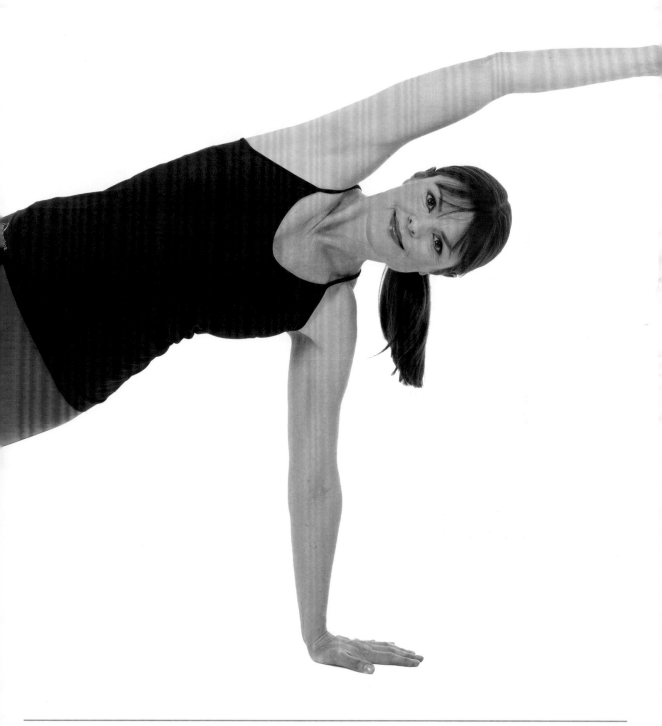

PILATES KIT

These simple pieces of equipment will help you get even more from your workouts

All you need to practise Pilates is your body and your mind! However, a few pieces of clothing and equipment can help support your body and ensure you get the maximum results from your workouts.

Ideally, you'll have a Pilates or yoga mat but, if not, you can fold a blanket so you have some form of cushioning underneath you during the floor exercises. Make sure you have enough space to move freely and wear comfortable, breathable clothing.

I've tried to keep things as simple as possible in this book so have chosen to use just a couple of pieces of useful, affordable kit for some of the moves. The first is a resistance or flex band. This simple but effective tool adds resistance to your exercises to increase the challenge and build your strength. Widely available, resistance bands come in three different strengths. I recommend selecting a medium resistance band for these exercises. However, if you're recovering from a shoulder injury, begin with a gentle resistance band.

A couple of the exercises use dumbbells to increase resistance. If you don't have any, you can use small bottles of water or cans of beans. Alternatively, you can simply imagine that you're using weights! It sounds silly, but try doing a bicep curl with an imaginary weight right now. Imagine you're lifting a really heavy bag on to your shoulder and you'll feel your muscles work much harder than doing the same thing without using your imagination.

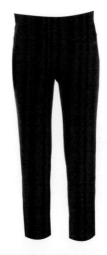

PILATES PANTS
For ease of movement, look for well-fitting pants in a stretchable fabric that won't ride up or down during the moves.
3/4 leggings, £12.50; usapro.co.uk

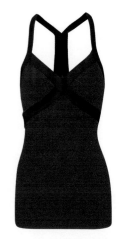

PILATES TANK
Choose something comfortable that allows movement without falling down.
Cross it tank, £59.95; wellicious.com

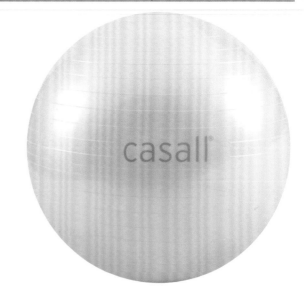

casall

GYM BALL
Not essential for this book but the wobble of a ball forces your core to work harder during exercises.
Casall gym ball, £24.95; simplysweat.com

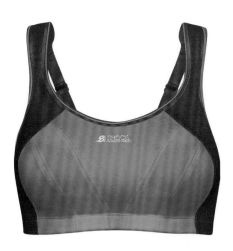

SPORTS BRA
A well-fitting sports bra is a must for every workout.
Active Flexi Wire, £28; shockabsorber.co.uk

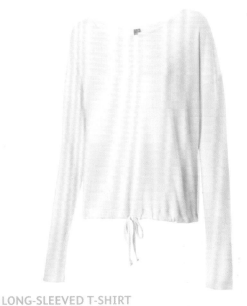

LONG-SLEEVED T-SHIRT
Your body temperature can vary during your workouts so have a
cover-up on hand to keep you warm.
Barbican long-sleeve yoga tee, £55; sweatybetty.com

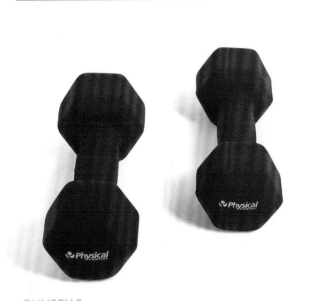

DUMBELLS
A basic set of hand weights costs less than £30. Choose a light weight
to avoid straining your neck during exercises.
Physical dumbells, from £5.50; physicalcompany.co.uk

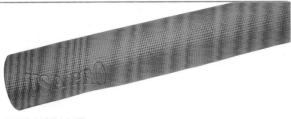

EXERCISE MAT
A mat is essential to protect your spine during the floor exercises.
Look for a non-slip mat.
Exercise mat, £6.99; store.usapro.co.uk

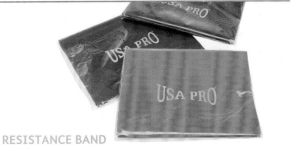

RESISTANCE BAND
These bands increase the challenge and effectiveness of your moves.
Body band, £5.99; store.usapro.co.uk

WARM UP

Before you begin your Pilates exercises you need to prepare your body so a good warm up is essential. Don't skimp, it won't take long

This warm up is designed to prime and prepare your whole body for exercise, increasing blood flow to your muscles and warming up your joints. Please don't skip the warm up, it will only take a couple of minutes. If it's cold, you're just out of bed or are feeling a little stiff, it's a great idea to repeat the circuit twice. If you have plenty of time, you could follow these moves with the basic exercises on page 26 for a more comprehensive warm up.

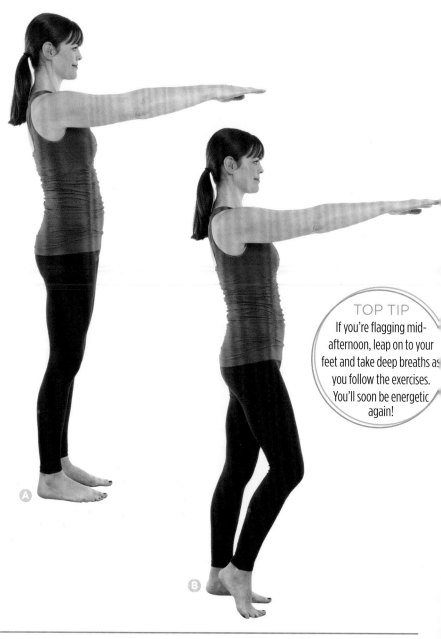

STANDING TIP-TOE MARCH

● Stand with your feet and knees hip-width apart.
● Keeping your shoulders down away from your ears, lift your arms out to shoulder height (A).
● Lift up high on to tip-toe. Now 'march' lowering alternate heels to the floor for 20 reps (B).

TOP TIP
If you're flagging mid-afternoon, leap on to your feet and take deep breaths as you follow the exercises. You'll soon be energetic again!

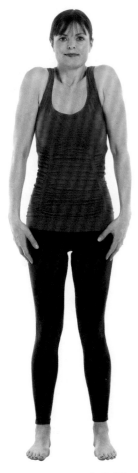

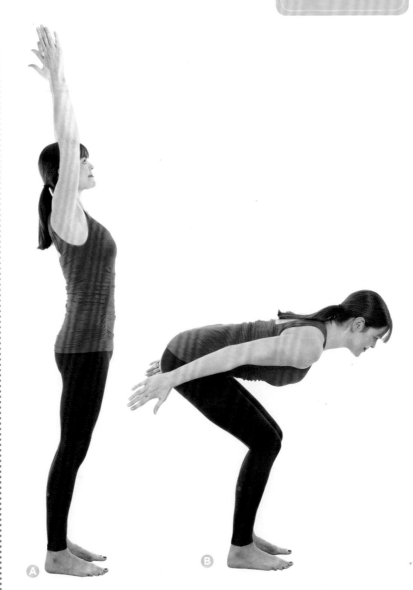

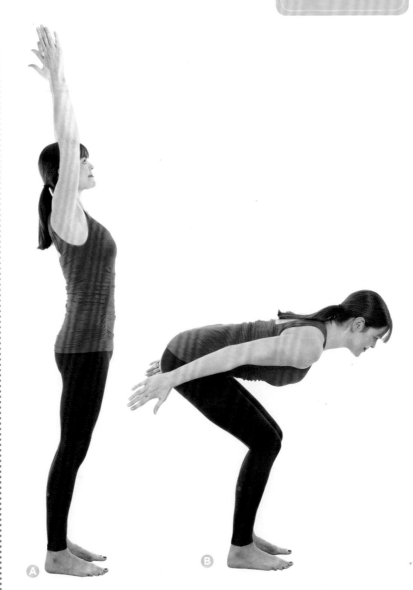

SHOULDER CIRCLES

● Stand with a tall posture and neutral spine.
● Circle your shoulders backwards 10 times, finishing with them open and your shoulder blades drawn gently back and down.

SKIING

● Stay standing as in the exercise opposite. Inhale to reach your arms up high overhead (A).
● Exhale to bend your hips and knees into a skiing position, swinging your arms back behind you (B).
● Inhale and reach arms back up overhead.
● Continue in time with your breath for 20 reps.

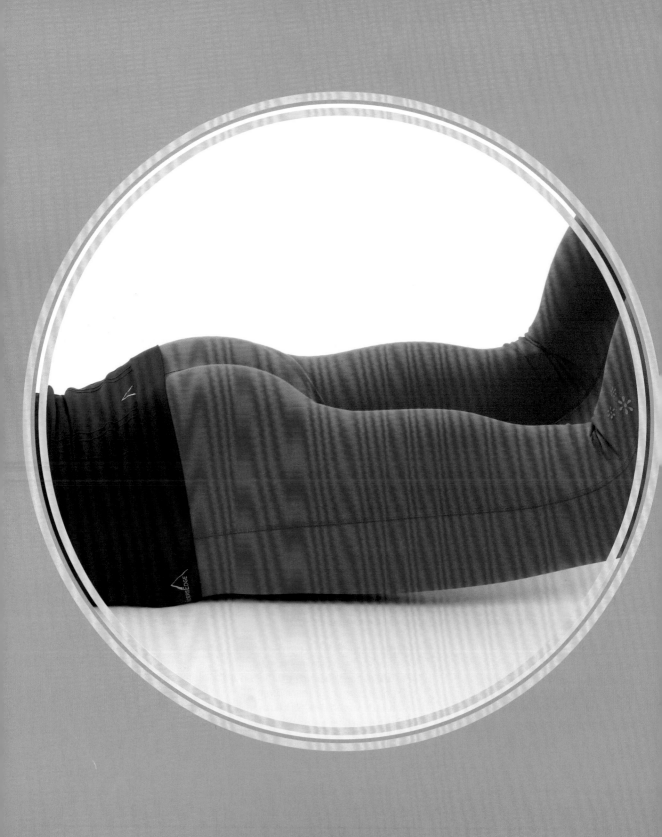

TONE YOUR BUM

✳ Your bottom contains one of the largest muscles in your body – the gluteus maximus. Known as a 'global' muscle, it's responsible for creating movement. Beneath it are lesser known muscles, called 'local' or 'stabiliser' muscles that help stabilise your pelvis. Pilates works both global and local muscles, helping your body to move as nature intended and keeping it strong and balanced with a firm bottom as a bonus!

Sitting on your behind for a large part of the day can create a weak and flabby bot. Pilates can help prevent this. For a strong and functioning behind, focus on each movement and think about the muscle that's working.

These exercises work on strengthening your glutes and hamstrings as well as the stabiliser muscles of your bottom and hips. Pay attention to the training tips since a very simple adjustment, such as rotating your foot and leg outwards, will make a big difference to the results.

INSIDE...

Crab walk

Oyster 1 & 2

Single leg bridge

Heel squeeze prone

Reverse kick

10-minute workout

CRAB WALK

Benefits: strengthens and sculpts
your outer hips and bottom

● Stand with your feet and knees
hip-width apart. Tie a band around your
legs just above your ankles ensuring there
is no slack in this position (A). Place your
hands on your hips and draw your
shoulders back and down.
● Take 10 steps to the right, keeping your
upper body still – no rocking (B)!
● Take 10 steps back to the left.
● Now rotate your legs outwards so that
your toes point out to the sides and
repeat 10 steps each way (C).
● Finally rotate your legs inwards so
that your toes turn in and repeat 10 steps
each way (D).
● As you get stronger, and if time allows,
you can perform two to three sets
of each of the exercises.

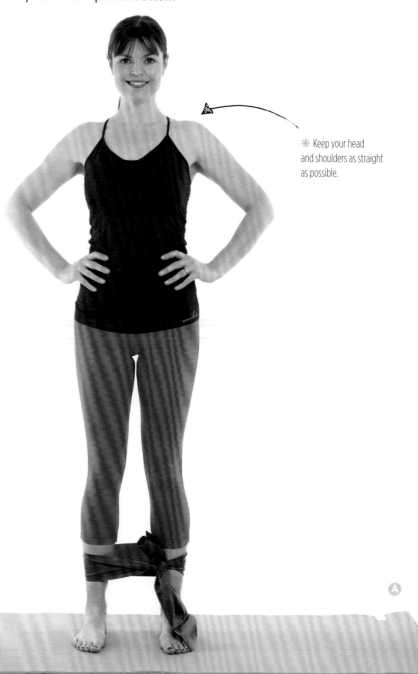

✳ Keep your head
and shoulders as straight
as possible.

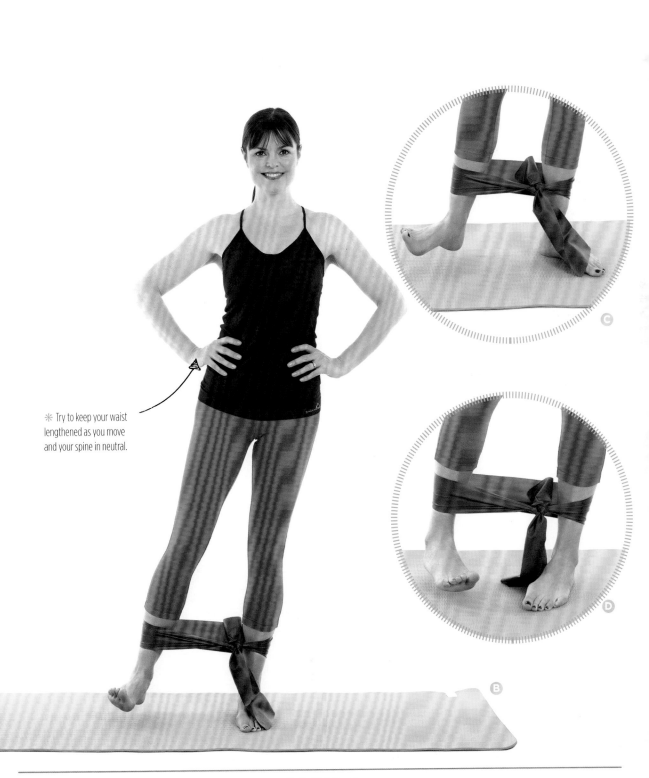

✳ Try to keep your waist lengthened as you move and your spine in neutral.

OYSTER 1 & 2

Benefits: strengthens and tightens your hips
and bottom and stabilises your pelvis

Part 1

● Lie on your right side, with your head
on your outstretched arm and both
knees bent (A).
● Exhale, engage navel to spine and open
your left knee – like a book opening
– keeping your hips still and stacked (B).
● Inhale to close.
● Repeat 12 times.

※ Keep your hips stacked
one on top of the other.

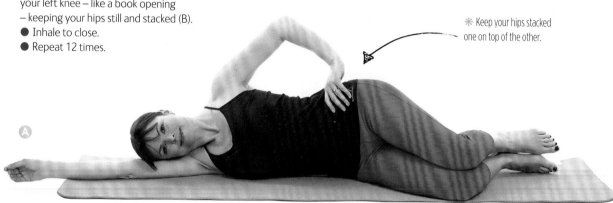

Ⓐ

※ Make sure that your
top hip stays completely
still as you open.

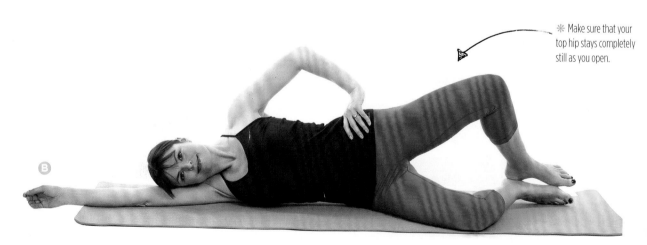

Ⓑ

※ Keep your core engaged so that
the weight of your waist is slightly
drawn off the floor.

Part 2
● Now repeat the same exercise but this time lift both feet off the floor with each repetition (C).
● Complete 12 repetitions.
● Now change to your left side and repeat part 1 and 2 on your right leg.

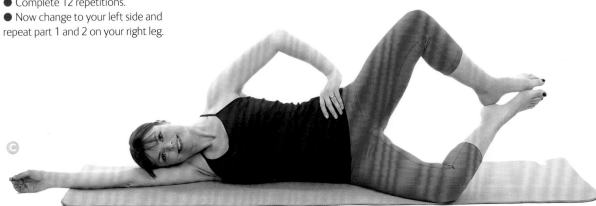

TO PROGRESS
● Tie the flex band around your knees with just a little slack in the closed position.
● Repeat the steps above against the resistance of the band.

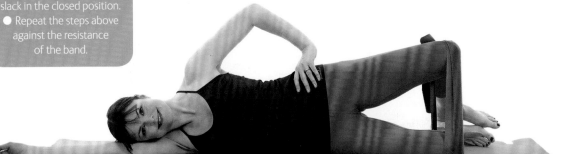

SINGLE LEG BRIDGE

Benefits: strengthens your glutes, hamstrings and pelvic stabilisers and balances your hip joints

● Lie on your back with your feet and knees hip-width apart (A).
● Exhale, engage navel to spine and use your glutes to lift your hips up in the air so that you form a straight line from your knee to hip to shoulder (B).
● Inhale, and keep a neutral spine and your pelvis level.
● Exhale to lift one foot off the floor (C). Inhale to place it back down maintaining a level pelvis throughout.
● Work alternate sides for 10 reps each.

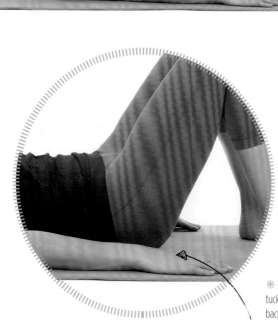

* Keep your tailbone slightly tucked under to prevent your lower back from arching.

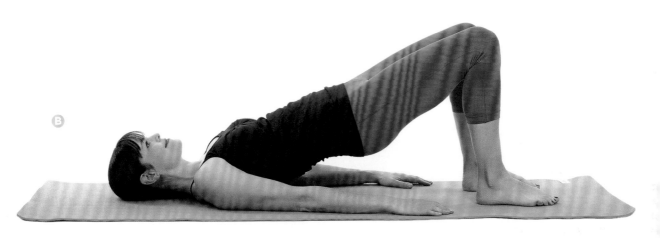

B

TO PROGRESS
- Lift your hips up as before and then lift your right leg to a table top (C).
- Lower and lift your hips up and down eight to 10 times working the left glute/hamstring.
- Replace your foot to the floor and lower your hips back down.
- Repeat on the other side for eight to 10 times.

✳ Imagine you have a spirit level on your hips to help you stay level.

✳ If you feel that your hamstring might cramp, stop and stretch (page 36).

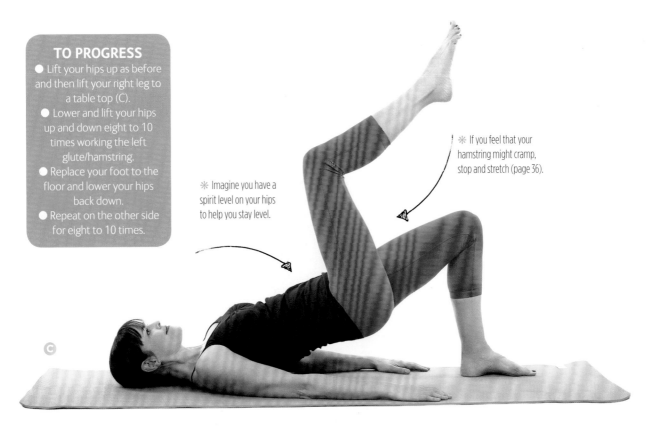

C

HEEL SQUEEZE PRONE
Benefits: lifts and tightens your bottom

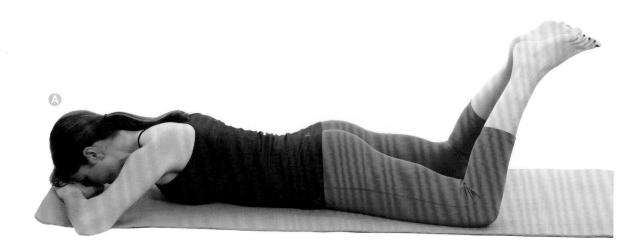

- Lie face down with your forehead supported on the back of your hands.
- Take your legs wide apart and bend your knees, bringing your heels together like a frog's legs (A).
- Keep your spine in neutral by slightly tucking your tailbone under by pressing your pubic bone into the mat and keep your core engaged.
- Inhale to prepare.
- Exhale and squeeze your heels together, squeezing your bottom tightly (B).
- Repeat eight long, slow breaths.
- To increase the intensity, lengthen your knees off the floor as you squeeze (C).

✳ Keep your spine in neutral throughout, and your abdominals drawn in.

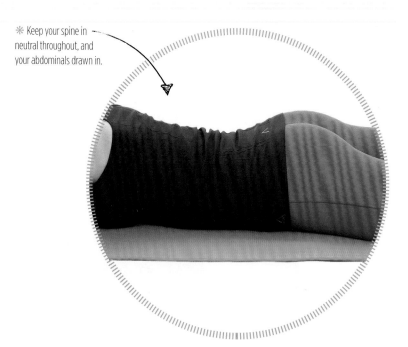

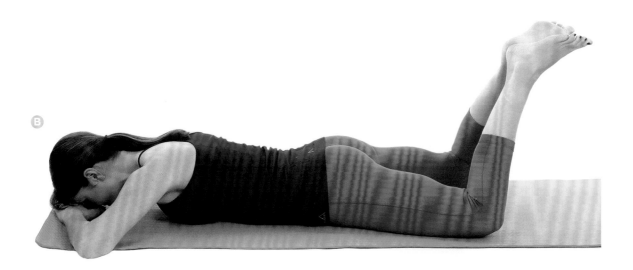

✳ Think of lengthening through the front of your thighs as you squeeze.

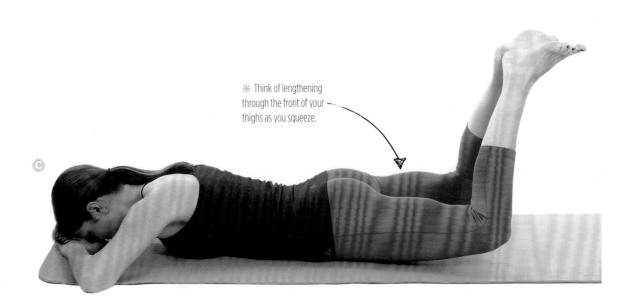

REVERSE KICK

Benefits: tightens and tones your bottom and
hamstrings and strengthens your shoulders and core

● Come on to all fours, then lower down
on to your elbows. Your elbows should be
under your shoulders and your knees
under your hips (A).
● Keeping your shoulders away from your
ears, draw navel to spine and straighten
out your left leg.
● Inhale to prepare.
● Exhale and use your bottom and
hamstrings to lift your left leg, keeping
your spine in neutral (B).
● Lift and lower your leg 12 times and on
the last repetition hold your leg in the up
position and pulse 12 times.
● Now bend the left leg and exhale to
press the sole of the foot up towards the
ceiling 12 times (C).
● Repeat on the right leg.

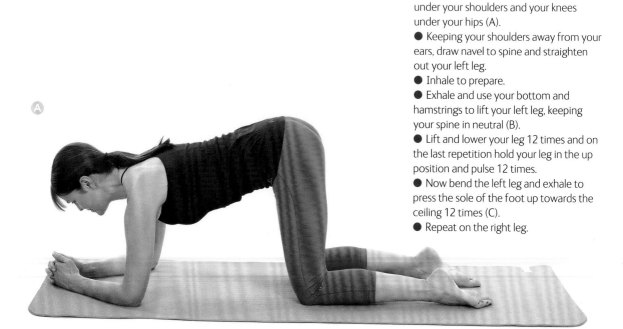

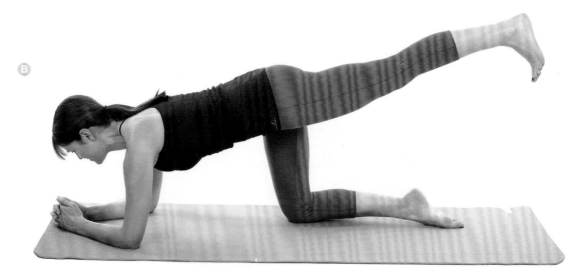

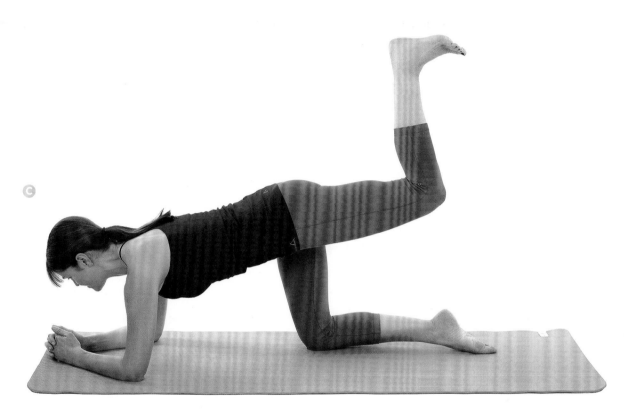

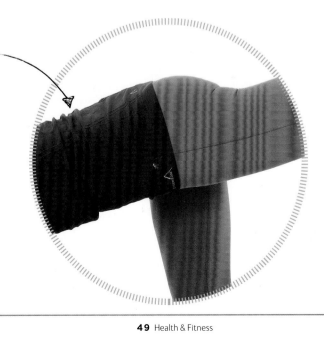

✳ Keep your abdominals drawn in and your spine in neutral throughout. Try to keep your knee straight and think of lifting from your bottom.

10-MINUTE BUM WORKOUT

Strengthen, tighten and tone your bottom, hips and
hamstrings with this speedy circuit

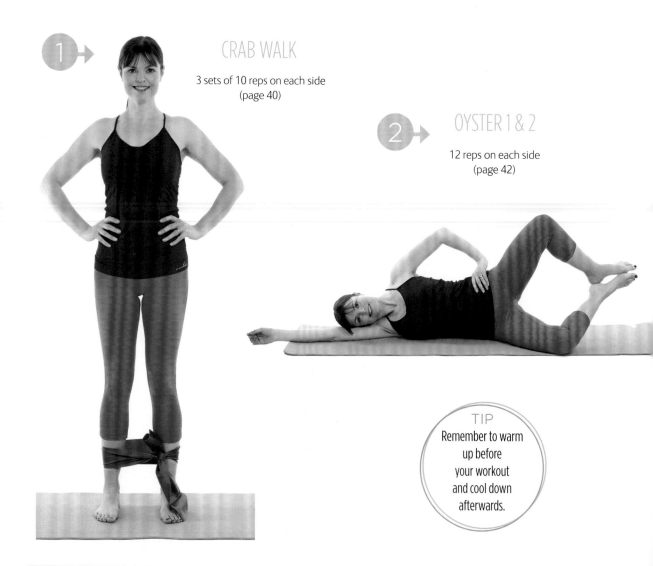

1 → CRAB WALK

3 sets of 10 reps on each side
(page 40)

2 → OYSTER 1 & 2

12 reps on each side
(page 42)

TIP
Remember to warm
up before
your workout
and cool down
afterwards.

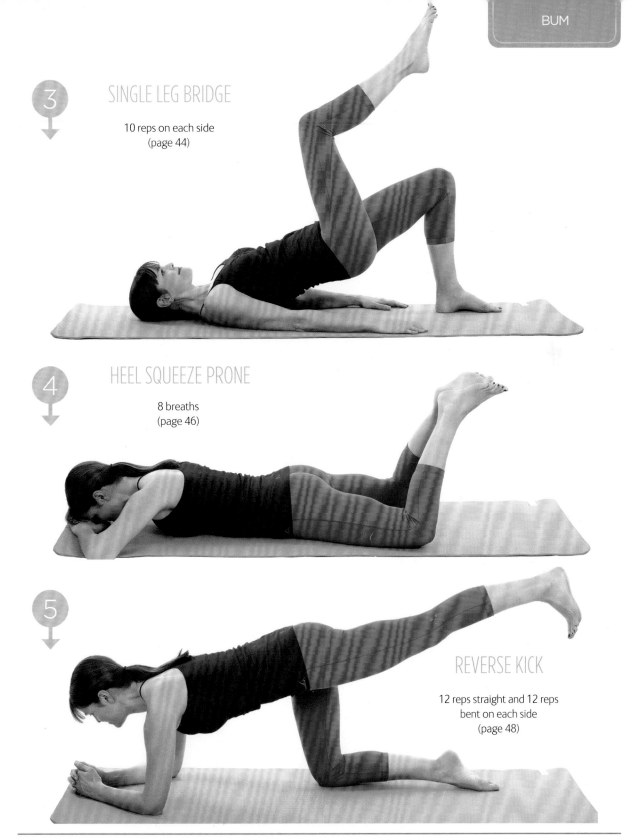

3 SINGLE LEG BRIDGE

10 reps on each side
(page 44)

4 HEEL SQUEEZE PRONE

8 breaths
(page 46)

5 REVERSE KICK

12 reps straight and 12 reps
bent on each side
(page 48)

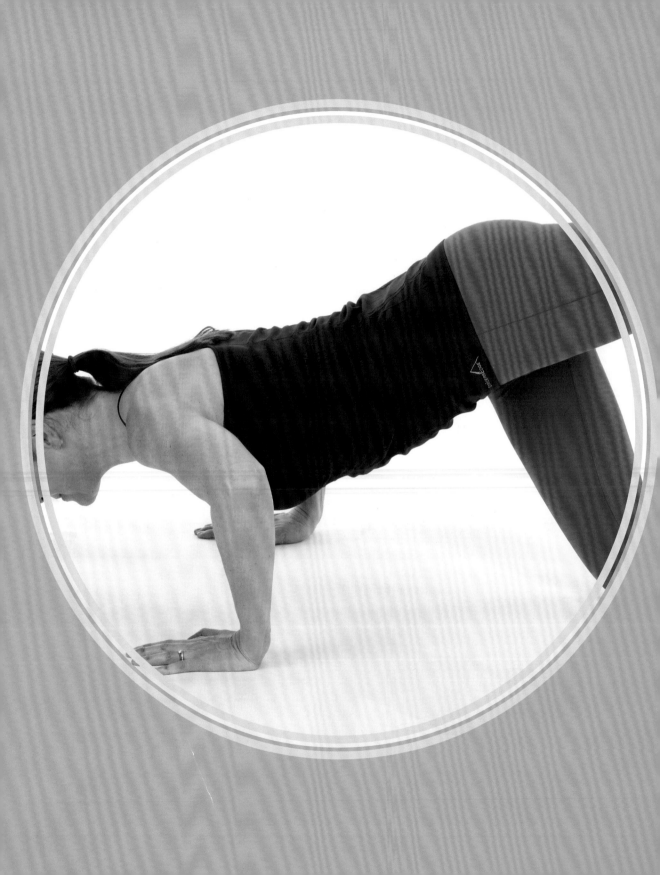

AMAZING ARMS

✳ Modern life is enough to give you a hunched back. Sitting at computers, hunching over portable devices or being in the car for hours on end is ageing us prematurely and giving us rounded shoulders and curved backs – not to mention headaches, stiff necks and sore shoulders!

This chapter focuses on counteracting these negative postures. You'll open your shoulders and chest, and lengthen and strengthen your upper back and shoulder muscles. We'll also target the global 'mover' muscles of the shoulders and arms to help create tone and definition. Goodbye bingo wings!

INSIDE...

Dumb waiter

Cat twist

Triceps with band

Arms ab curl

Controlled push up

Half roll back with biceps curl

10-minute workout

DUMB WAITER

Benefits: strengthens your shoulder postural
muscles and opens your chest

● Stand with feet hip-width apart, elbows touching your waist and bent to a right angle with your palms facing up.
● Exhale and gently draw your navel in towards your spine (A).
● Inhale as you slowly move your hands apart while working the muscles between your shoulder blades. Keep your forearms parallel to the floor throughout (B).
● Exhale to move your hands back to the start position.
● Repeat eight times.

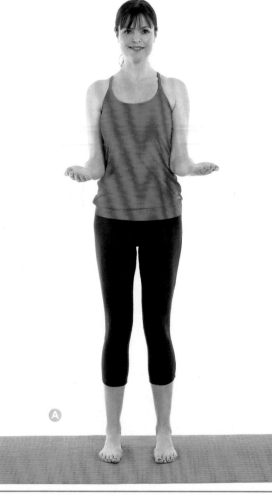

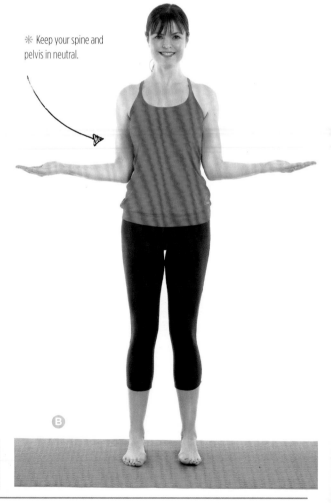

✳ Keep your spine and pelvis in neutral.

TO PROGRESS

● Hold one end of a flex band in each hand (A) and exhale to gently pull against the band (B). Keep the movement as smooth as possible.

✳ Try to keep your shoulders down throughout, with a gentle abdominal engagement.

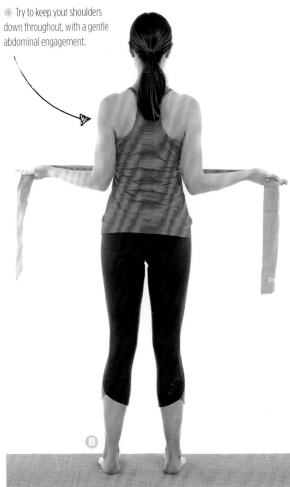

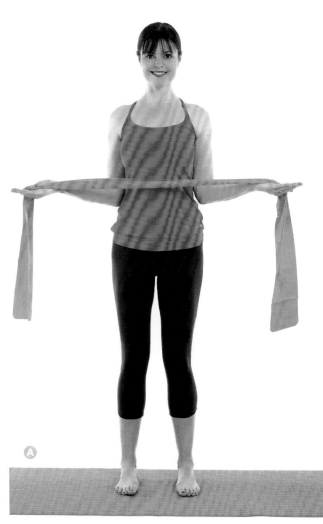

Ⓐ

Ⓑ

✳ The aim is to locate the muscles around your shoulder blades.

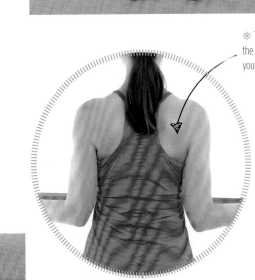

CAT TWIST

Benefits: strengthens and mobilises your shoulder girdle and upper back, and counteracts rounded shoulders

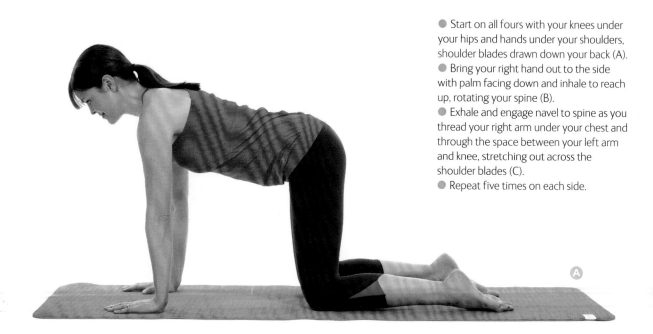

● Start on all fours with your knees under your hips and hands under your shoulders, shoulder blades drawn down your back (A).
● Bring your right hand out to the side with palm facing down and inhale to reach up, rotating your spine (B).
● Exhale and engage navel to spine as you thread your right arm under your chest and through the space between your left arm and knee, stretching out across the shoulder blades (C).
● Repeat five times on each side.

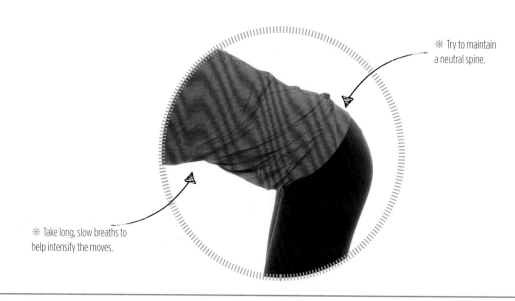

✳ Try to maintain a neutral spine.

✳ Take long, slow breaths to help intensify the moves.

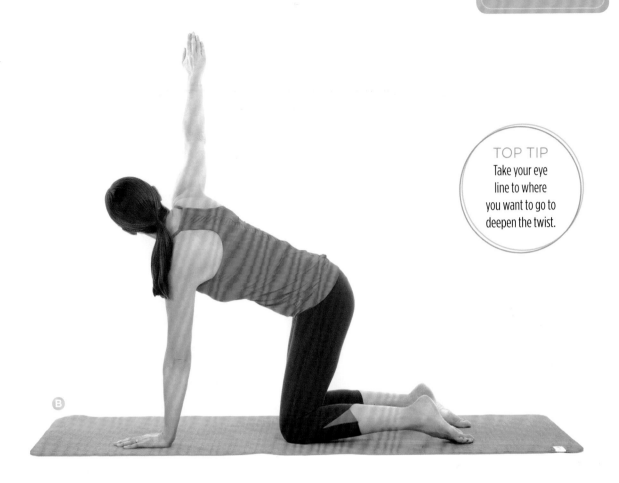

TOP TIP
Take your eye line to where you want to go to deepen the twist.

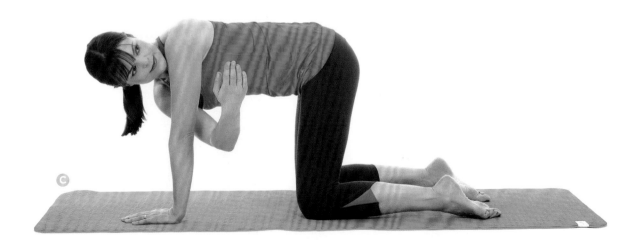

TRICEPS WITH BAND

Benefits: strengthens the back of
your upper arms and shoulders

● Kneel up – with a neutral spine – and
drop the flex band behind you with your
right arm.
● Take hold of the other end with your
left hand, ensuring there's some tension
in the band (A).
● Keeping your left hand firmly in the
small of your back, inhale to prepare.
● Exhale and straighten your right arm up
over your head, pulling on the band (B).
● Inhale and slowly bend your arm
back down.
● Repeat 12 times on each arm.

✳ Keep your eye-line
straight ahead and your
shoulders open.

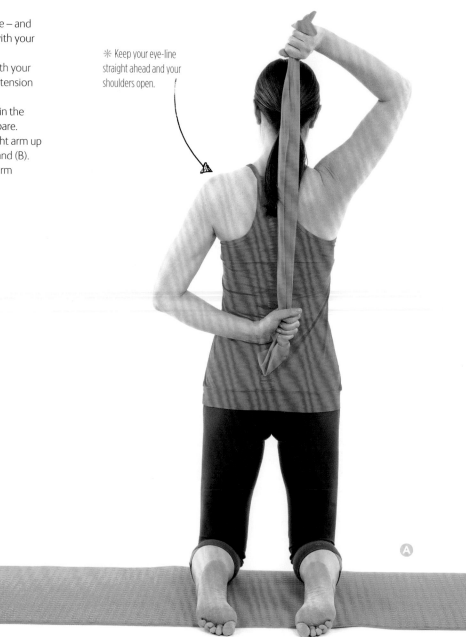

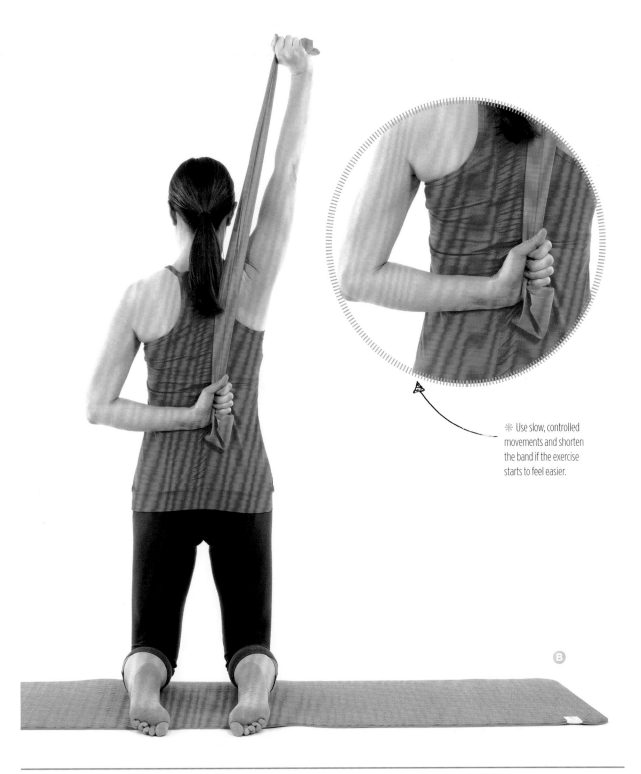

✳ Use slow, controlled movements and shorten the band if the exercise starts to feel easier.

Ⓑ

ARMS AB CURL

Benefits: strengthens the front and back of your
arms as well as your abs

● Lie on your back with your knees bent
and your feet and knees hip-width apart
with a light dumbbell or a bottle of water in
each hand (A).
● Exhale, engage navel to spine and curl
your head and shoulders off the mat,
lifting your arms off the floor with a
slightly bent elbow (B).
● Keep your head and shoulders up as you
exhale to bend your elbows, bringing the
weights towards your shoulders (C).
● Inhale to straighten.

● Do this 10 times.
● Bring your head and arms back to the
floor and rest for a few breath cycles.
● Now exhale and lift your head and
shoulders again, this time bringing your
arms straight up towards the ceiling (D).
● Keeping your head and shoulders up,
bend your elbows, lowering the weights
down towards your ears (E).
● Do this 10 times.
● Return to the floor and gently roll your
head from side to side to relax your neck.

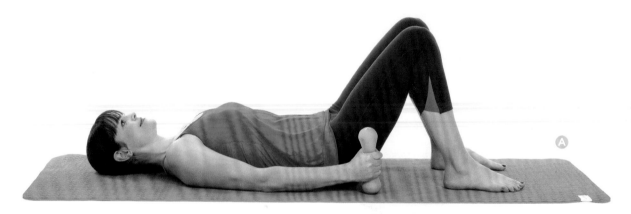

✳ Keep your shoulders
away from your ears and
your shoulder blades
drawn down your back.

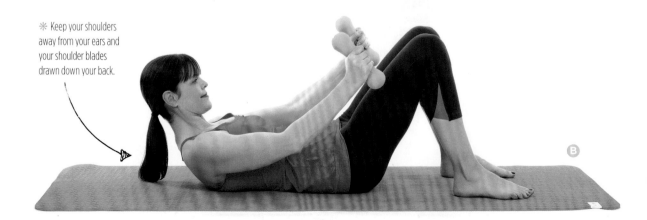

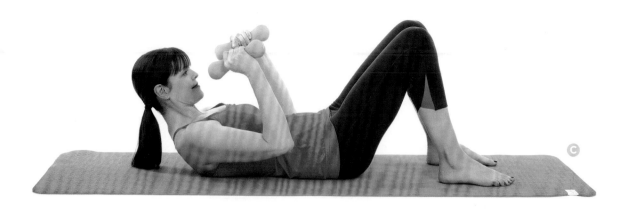

※ If you feel this is too challenging for your neck, support your head in one hand and work one arm at a time or support your head on a cushion and work both arms.

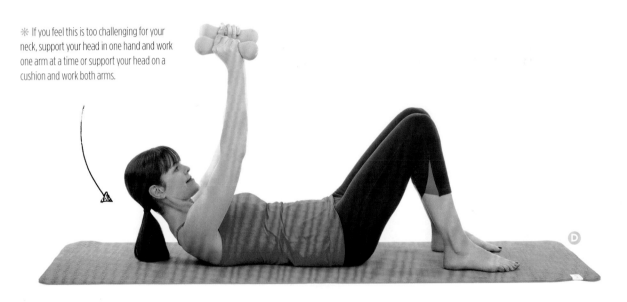

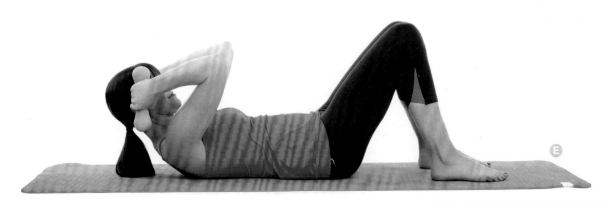

CONTROLLED PUSH UP

Benefits: strengthens and sculpts the muscles
of your chest, shoulders and arms

- Kneel on all fours with your feet and knees hips-width apart.
- Extend your left leg out behind you with your foot at hip height (A).
- Inhale as you slowly lower your chest down between your hands keeping your elbows close by your sides and pointing straight back while your leg raises (B).
- Exhale, engage navel to spine and press back up.
- Repeat eight to 10 times then do a second set with your right leg extended.

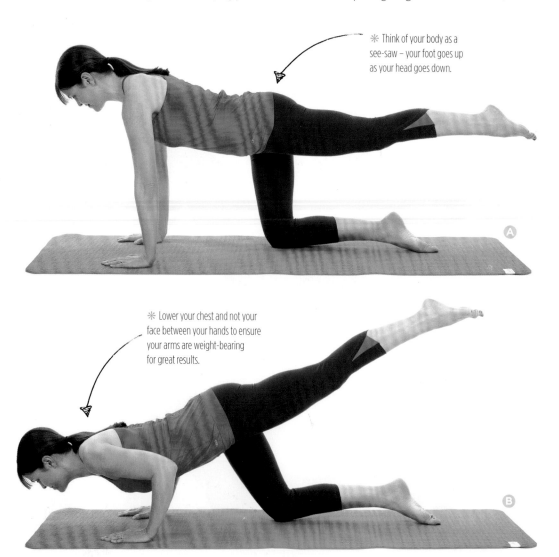

✳ Think of your body as a see-saw – your foot goes up as your head goes down.

✳ Lower your chest and not your face between your hands to ensure your arms are weight-bearing for great results.

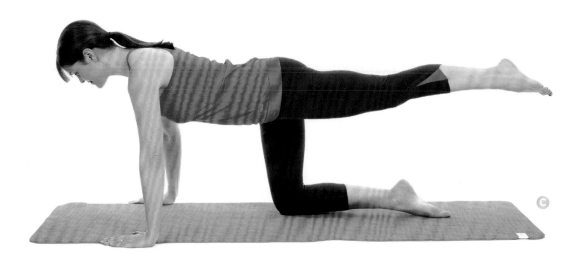

✳ Keep your abdominals drawn in and your back straight.

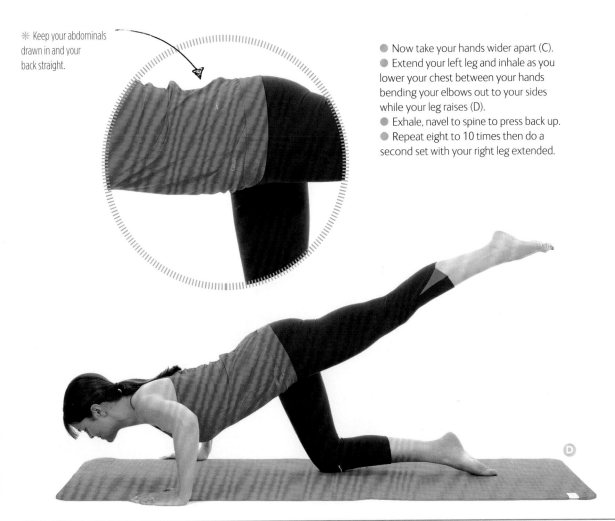

● Now take your hands wider apart (C).
● Extend your left leg and inhale as you lower your chest between your hands bending your elbows out to your sides while your leg raises (D).
● Exhale, navel to spine to press back up.
● Repeat eight to 10 times then do a second set with your right leg extended.

HALF ROLL BACK WITH BICEPS CURL
Benefits: tones the front of your arms
while strengthening your abs

- Sit up with your knees bent and a flex band wrapped around your toes.
- Hold the flex band in your fists with your thumbs pointing up and the ends of the band passing out through your thumbs (A).
- Inhale to prepare.
- Then exhale, engage navel to spine and tuck your tailbone under as you roll half way back (B).
- Hold this position, keeping your abs firmly in, your shoulders back and down and your lumbar spine in a 'C' shape.
- Now perform 12 biceps curls, exhaling to pull on the band and bringing your thumbs towards your shoulders (C).
- Finish by sitting up tall with your shoulders back and down.

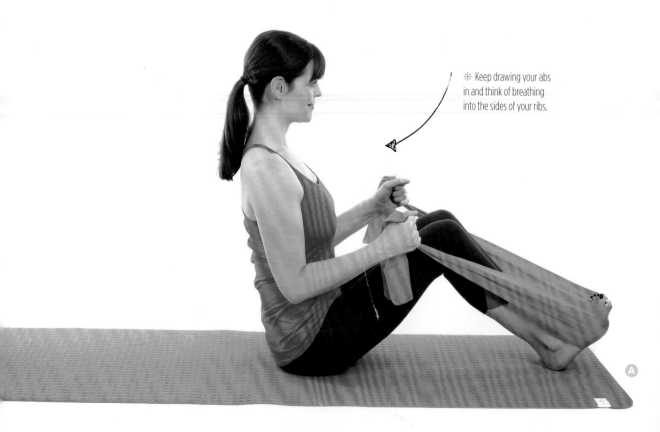

✳ Keep drawing your abs in and think of breathing into the sides of your ribs.

A

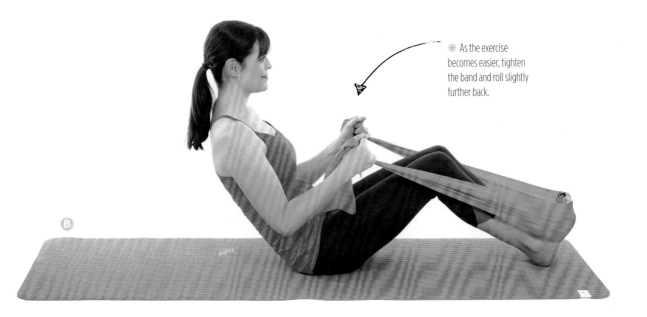

B

✳ As the exercise becomes easier, tighten the band and roll slightly further back.

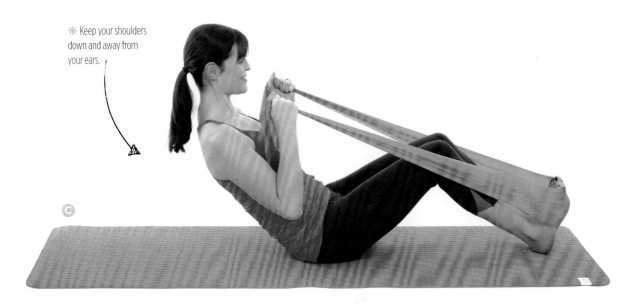

✳ Keep your shoulders down and away from your ears.

C

10-MINUTE ARMS WORKOUT

Tone your arms, open your chest and improve
your posture with this fab upper body workout

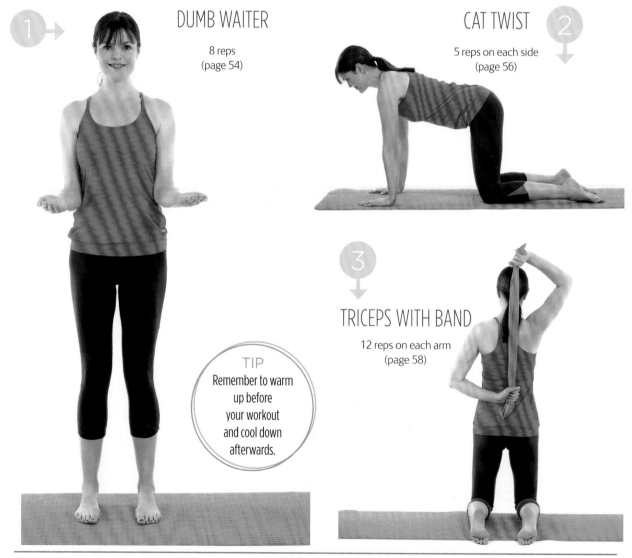

1 ➤ DUMB WAITER

8 reps
(page 54)

CAT TWIST **2** ↓

5 reps on each side
(page 56)

3 ↓

TRICEPS WITH BAND

12 reps on each arm
(page 58)

TIP
Remember to warm
up before
your workout
and cool down
afterwards.

4 ARMS AB CURL

10 reps biceps
10 reps triceps
(page 60)

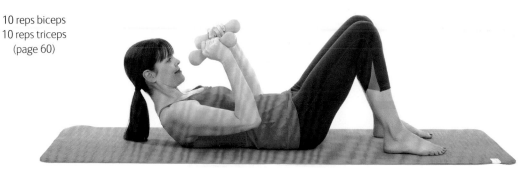

5 CONTROLLED PUSH UP

8-10 reps,
both narrow and wide
(page 62)

6 ROLL BACK BICEPS CURL

12 reps
(page 64)

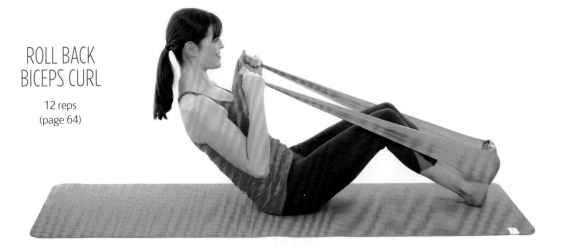

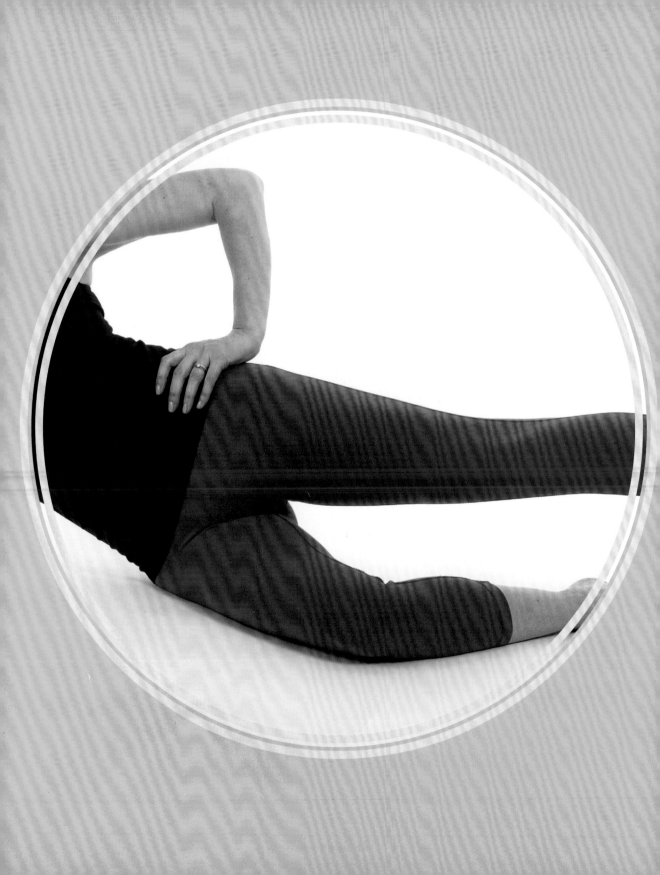

LEAN LEGS

This chapter is all about creating the illusion of longer, leaner legs. You can't make your legs longer than you were blessed with but, by improving your posture and exercising the right way, you can make yourself look taller and you can slim your hips and thighs to enhance the effect.

These exercises only use the weight of your body so they tighten and tone rather than build your muscles. They work on both the large 'global' muscles of the hips and thighs, and the smaller 'local' muscles, helping to tighten and pull up in your buttocks and outer hips.

You'll often be asked to 'lengthen and lift' the legs instead of 'lift'. This is important. Take, for example, the side leg lift exercise (page 74). Try lying on your side and just lift and lower the leg. Now perform the exercise following the instructions and teaching tips carefully, lengthening your leg from the waist to the toe – just feel the difference it makes!

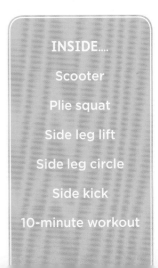

INSIDE....

Scooter

Plie squat

Side leg lift

Side leg circle

Side kick

10-minute workout

SCOOTER

Benefits: strengthens your hip and buttock on your standing leg, improves your balance and core strength and strengthens and tones your thighs

✳ Keep your stationary knee completely still with it over and in line with your second toe.

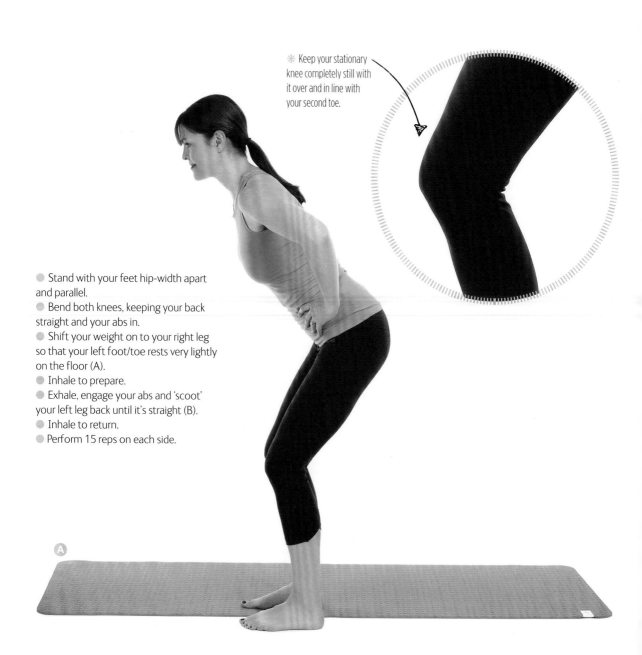

● Stand with your feet hip-width apart and parallel.
● Bend both knees, keeping your back straight and your abs in.
● Shift your weight on to your right leg so that your left foot/toe rests very lightly on the floor (A).
● Inhale to prepare.
● Exhale, engage your abs and 'scoot' your left leg back until it's straight (B).
● Inhale to return.
● Perform 15 reps on each side.

Ⓐ

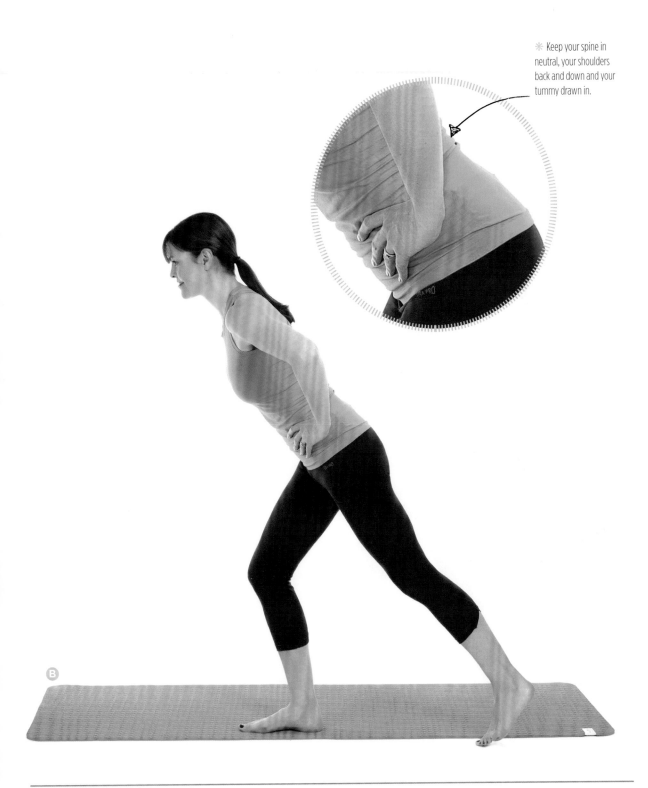

✳ Keep your spine in neutral, your shoulders back and down and your tummy drawn in.

Ⓑ

PLIÉ SQUAT

Benefits: shapes and lifts your bottom and works your inner thighs

● Stand with your feet wide apart and your toes pointing outwards.
● Place your hands on your hips and draw your shoulders back and down (A).
● Inhale and bend your knees out wide over your toes (B).
● Exhale and squeeze your bottom as you push yourself back upright.
● Repeat this 15 times.
● Now hold in the 'down' position and lift your heels up and down 10 times (C).
● For more intensity, hold dumbbells in front of your thighs and lift them straight out to shoulder height with each plié.

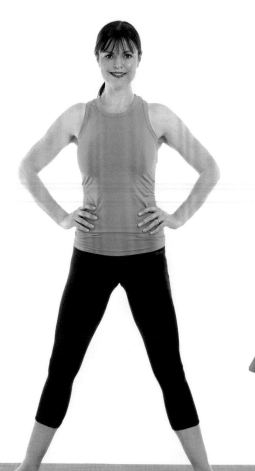

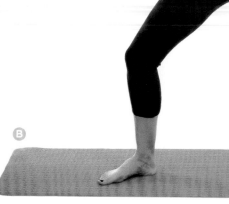

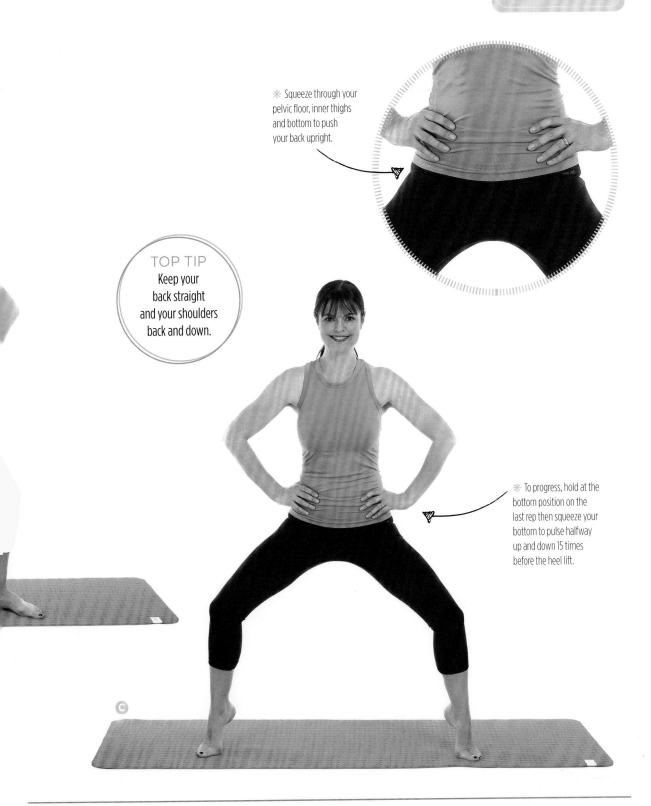

✳ Squeeze through your pelvic floor, inner thighs and bottom to push your back upright.

TOP TIP
Keep your back straight and your shoulders back and down.

✳ To progress, hold at the bottom position on the last rep then squeeze your bottom to pulse halfway up and down 15 times before the heel lift.

C

SIDE LEG LIFT

Benefits: strengthens and sculpts
your outer hips and bottom

● Lie on your right side with your head on
your outstretched arm, your bottom leg
bent and top leg out straight and raised
slightly (A).

● Place your top hand on your hip and try
to lengthen your waist off the floor (B).

● Exhale to lift the top leg with your foot
parallel to the floor (C).

● Inhale to lower.

● Do this 10 times.

● Repeat the exercise 10 times with your
leg turned inwards and your toes pointing
towards the floor.

● Now repeat the exercise a further 10
times with your leg turned out and your
toes pointing up towards the ceiling (D).

TOP TIP
For best results, slowly
exhale and tighten
your invisible corset
each time you lift
your leg.

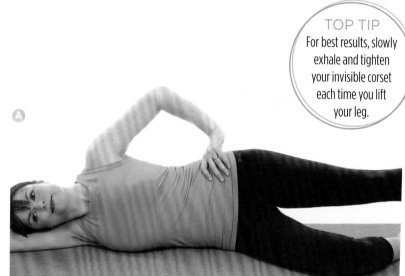

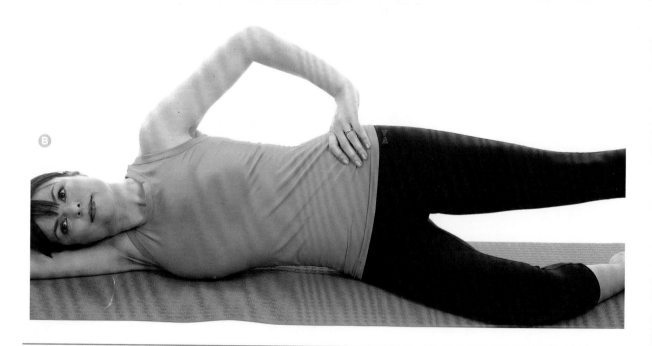

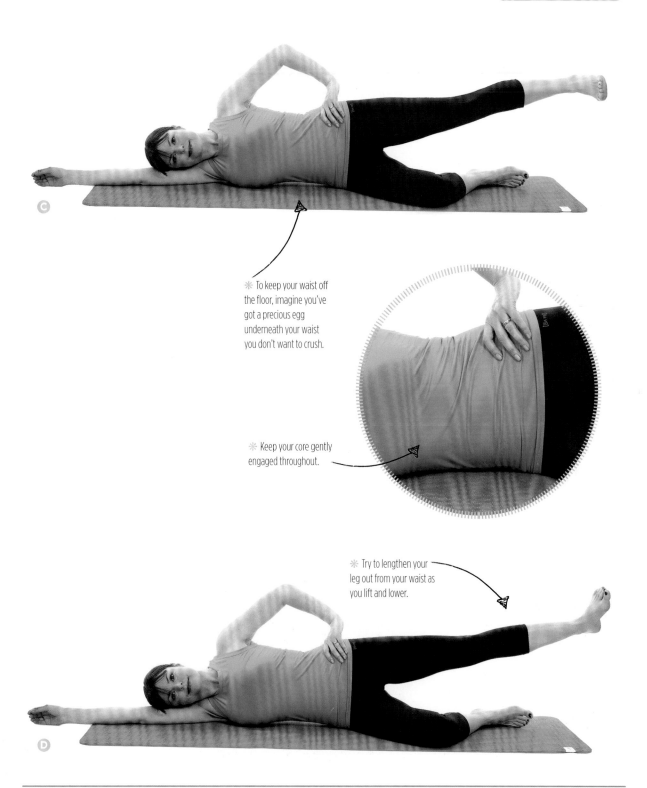

✳ To keep your waist off the floor, imagine you've got a precious egg underneath your waist you don't want to crush.

✳ Keep your core gently engaged throughout.

✳ Try to lengthen your leg out from your waist as you lift and lower.

C

D

SIDE LEG CIRCLE

Benefits: strengthens and sculpts
your outer hips and bottom

● Stay on your right side as in the
side leg lift on the previous page.
● This time instead of lifting your leg,
stretch it out long and circle it around
10 times in each direction (B).

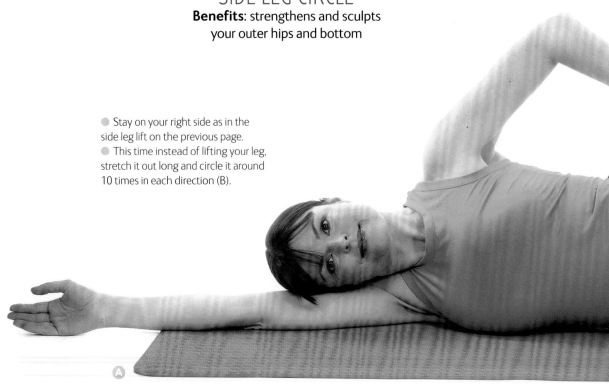

✳ Keep your waist lengthened off
the floor as with the side leg lift
and reach out as though you're
trying to trace the inside edge of
a barrel placed just out of reach
of your foot.

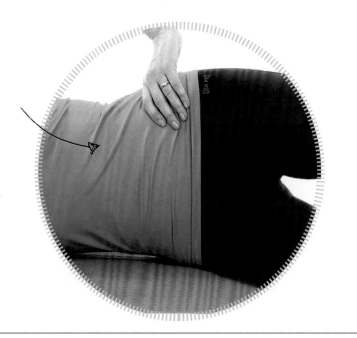

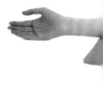

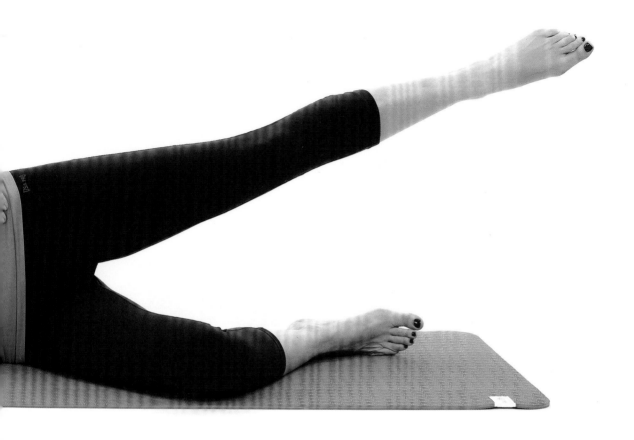

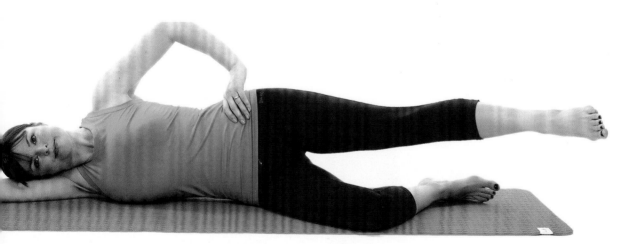

B

SIDE KICK

Benefits: strengthens and sculpts
your outer hips and bottom

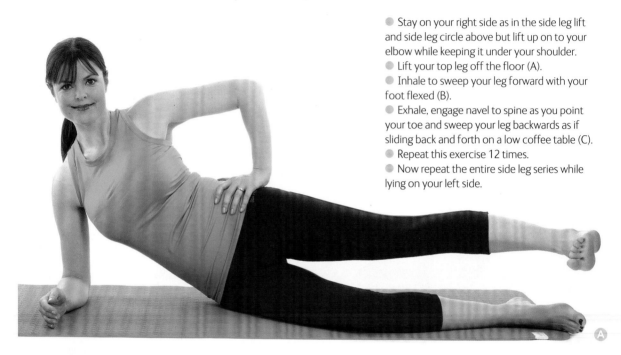

● Stay on your right side as in the side leg lift
and side leg circle above but lift up on to your
elbow while keeping it under your shoulder.
● Lift your top leg off the floor (A).
● Inhale to sweep your leg forward with your
foot flexed (B).
● Exhale, engage navel to spine as you point
your toe and sweep your leg backwards as if
sliding back and forth on a low coffee table (C).
● Repeat this exercise 12 times.
● Now repeat the entire side leg series while
lying on your left side.

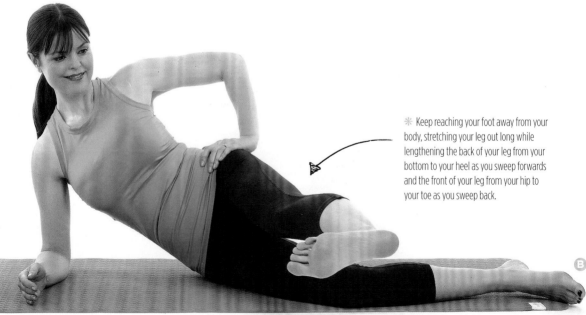

✳ Keep reaching your foot away from your
body, stretching your leg out long while
lengthening the back of your leg from your
bottom to your heel as you sweep forwards
and the front of your leg from your hip to
your toe as you sweep back.

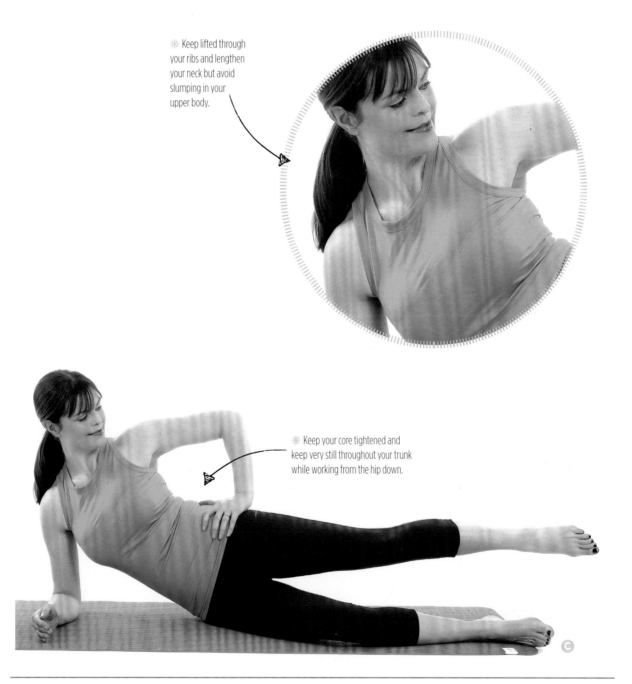

✳ Keep lifted through your ribs and lengthen your neck but avoid slumping in your upper body.

✳ Keep your core tightened and keep very still throughout your trunk while working from the hip down.

10-MINUTE LEG WORKOUT

Strengthen and tone your buttocks and outer hips,
and work your inner thighs with this leg workout

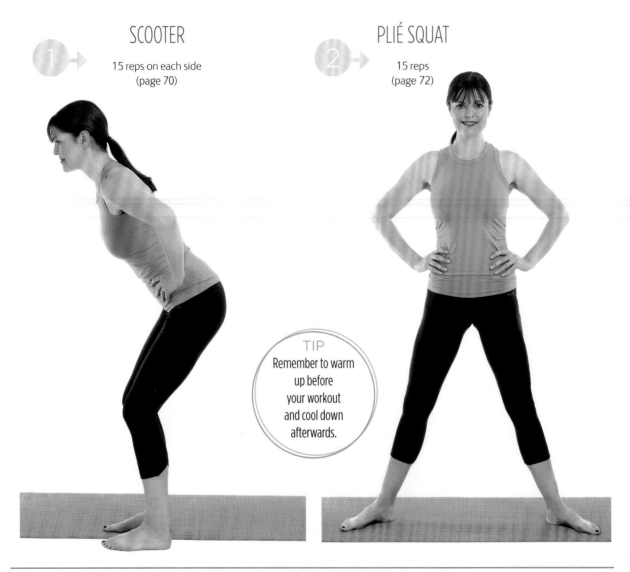

1 → SCOOTER

15 reps on each side
(page 70)

2 → PLIÉ SQUAT

15 reps
(page 72)

TIP
Remember to warm
up before
your workout
and cool down
afterwards.

3 SIDE LEG LIFT

3 sets of 10 reps
on each side
(page 74)

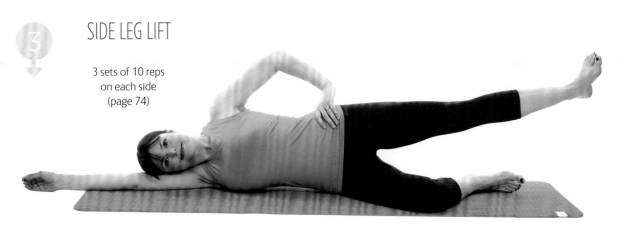

4 SIDE LEG CIRCLE

10 reps in each direction
on both sides
(page 76)

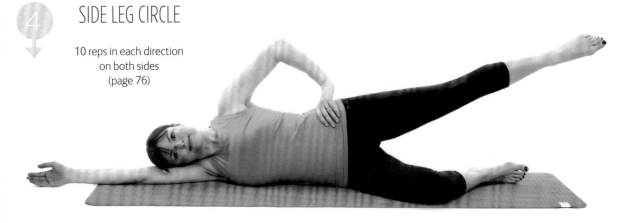

5 SIDE KICK

12 reps on each side
(page 78)

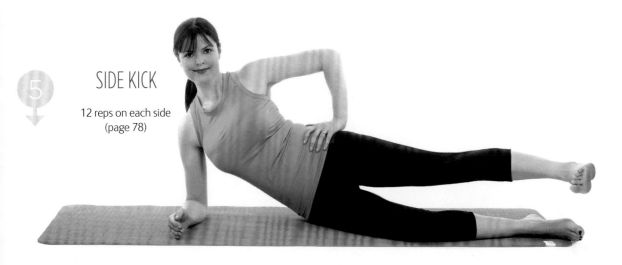

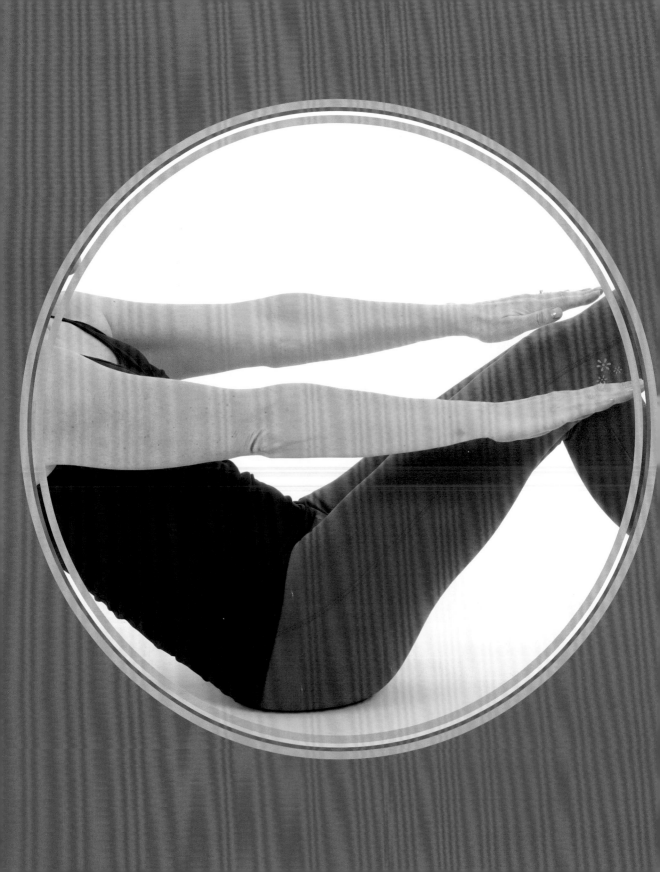

FLAT ABS

✳ When asked which part of their body they'd like to improve, many people say their abs, tummy, waist, love handles or muffin top. Our mid-sections are a problem area due to too much body fat, poor posture and weak tummy muscles. Pilates will not significantly reduce body fat – this is where a balanced routine with some cardiovascular exercise and a healthy diet are needed – but it will give you great abdominal tone, better posture and a flatter mid-section.

All Pilates exercises start by engaging your centre, so this book will help you work towards a stronger core and better abs. And, the more you practise Pilates, the more natural the moves will become until you use its principles in your everyday life and other sports you do, all enhancing the effect on your core.

INSIDE...

Roll up

Scissor legs

Criss-cross

Plank

Double leg stretch

10-minute workout

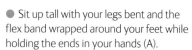

ROLL UP (BAND BEGINNERS)

Benefits: increases spine mobility and strengthens your abs

- Sit up tall with your legs bent and the flex band wrapped around your feet while holding the ends in your hands (A).
- Exhale and draw navel to spine as you tilt your pelvis and begin rolling half way back towards the floor (B).
- Inhale and roll back up keeping your abs drawn in.
- Repeat five to eight times.

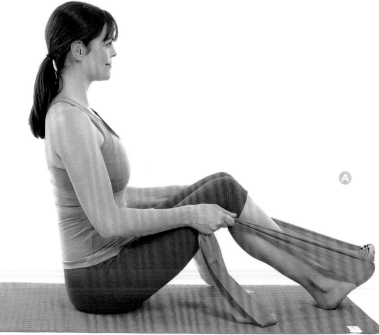

A

✳ Keep navel to spine throughout and your shoulders away from your ears.

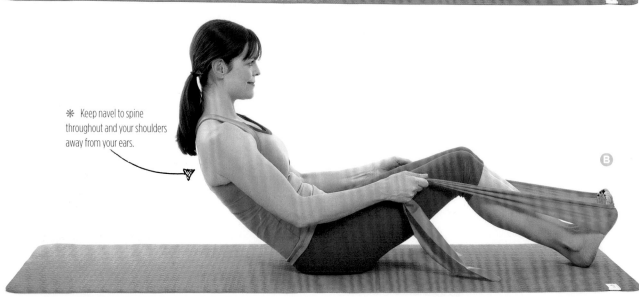

B

TOP TIP
Really use your breath here.
Slowly exhale through pursed
lips and don't hold your
breath through the
hard parts!

TO PROGRESS
● Sit with your legs out
straight in front of you and
the band around your feet (A).
● Proceed as opposite, then
inhale to prepare and exhale
to roll down with control until
you reach the floor (B).
● Inhale to stay down.
● Exhale and tuck your
tailbone under, drawing navel
to spine as you roll back up
one vertebra at a time.
● Repeat eight times.
● Once you can do this with
good control, repeat the steps
above without the band,
holding your arms out in front.

✱ Imagine your spine is
like a string of pearls. Lift
and lower one pearl – or
vertebra – at a time.

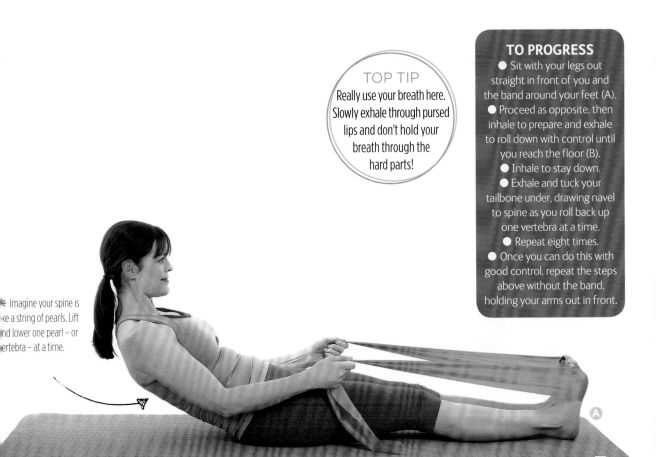

✱ If your feet try to lift off the
floor then go back a step and
focus more on your abs. Hold
the band tighter if you need to.

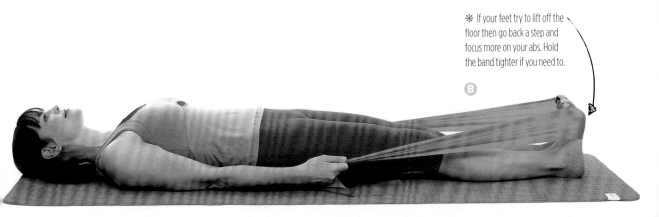

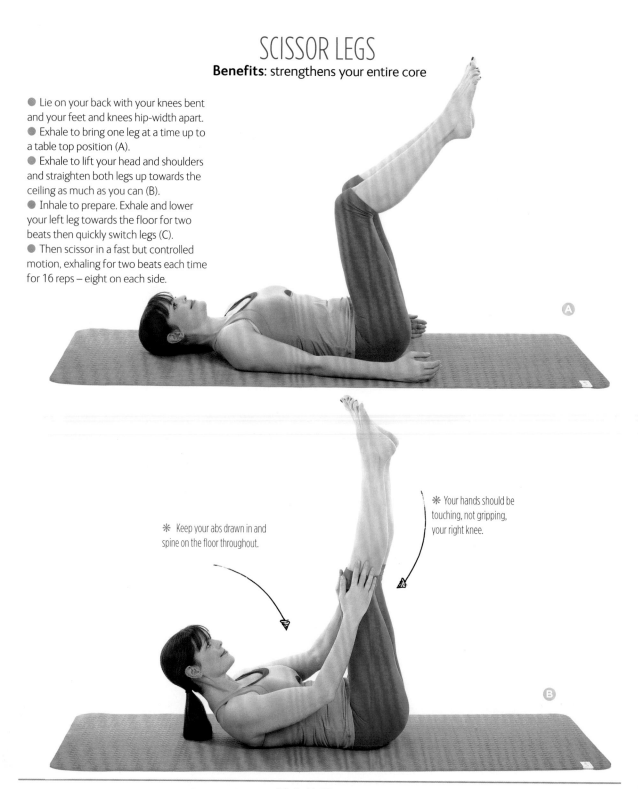

SCISSOR LEGS

Benefits: strengthens your entire core

● Lie on your back with your knees bent and your feet and knees hip-width apart.
● Exhale to bring one leg at a time up to a table top position (A).
● Exhale to lift your head and shoulders and straighten both legs up towards the ceiling as much as you can (B).
● Inhale to prepare. Exhale and lower your left leg towards the floor for two beats then quickly switch legs (C).
● Then scissor in a fast but controlled motion, exhaling for two beats each time for 16 reps – eight on each side.

A

✳ Keep your abs drawn in and spine on the floor throughout.

✳ Your hands should be touching, not gripping, your right knee.

B

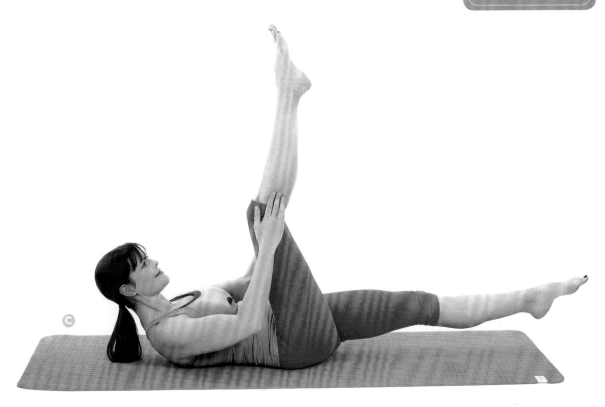

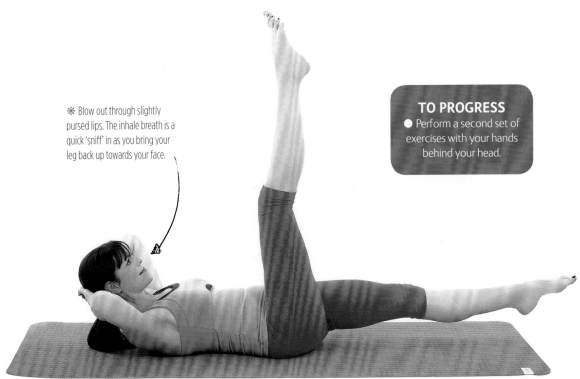

✳ Blow out through slightly pursed lips. The inhale breath is a quick 'sniff' in as you bring your leg back up towards your face.

TO PROGRESS
● Perform a second set of exercises with your hands behind your head.

CRISS-CROSS

Benefits: strengthens your core, particularly your oblique muscles, and tightens and tones your waist

● Lie on your back with your knees bent and hip-width apart.
● Exhale to bring one leg at a time up to the table-top position.
● Take your hands behind your head and exhale, engaging navel to spine to lift your head and shoulders off the floor (A).
● Inhale to prepare.
● Exhale and peel your left shoulder across towards your right hip as you extend your left leg out. Keep it as low as you can while keeping your stomach flat and your back flat and still (B).
● Inhale and move back to the centre then exhale in the opposite direction.
● Repeat 12 slow repetitions followed by 16 fast, but controlled reps.

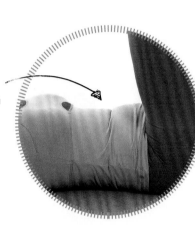

✳ Try to keep your stomach flat throughout and move in a controlled manner. Don't let your hips rock as you move.

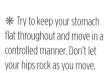

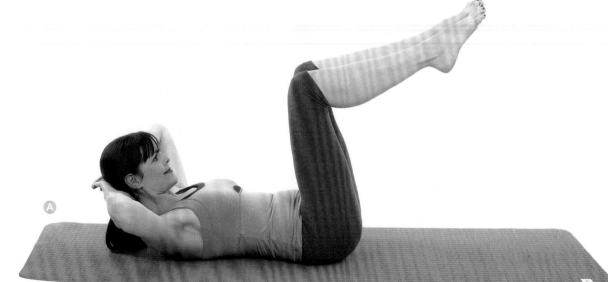

Ⓐ

BEGINNERS
● Keep both feet on the floor with your knees bent and draw your opposite shoulder to your hip 16 times.
● When this feels easier, keep both legs in a table top while criss-crossing your shoulders.
● Finally move on to the full exercise

✳ Keep your elbows wide and cross your shoulder, not elbow, towards your opposite hip.

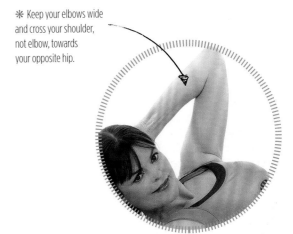

✳ Imagine you're folding your shoulder towards the opposite hip.

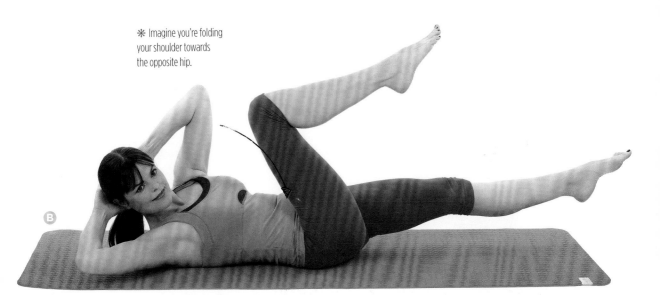

PLANK

Benefits: one of the best core exercises which flattens your abs and strengthens your entire torso

● Start on all fours with your hands under your shoulders and knees under your hips.
● Draw navel to spine and keep your back and hips still as you extend one leg at a time behind you to rest on your toes (A).
● Hold your body straight like a plank with your weight supported on your hands and toes (B).
● Start with a 20 second hold and build up to a minute or more.

✳ Build up gradually and always rest if you feel you're losing form.

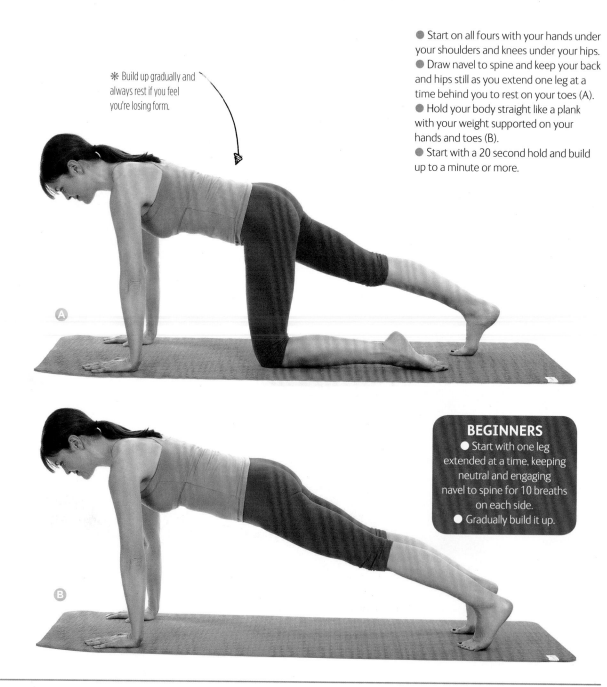

BEGINNERS
● Start with one leg extended at a time, keeping neutral and engaging navel to spine for 10 breaths on each side.
○ Gradually build it up.

TO PROGRESS
● As with the main exercise, but lift one foot from the floor at a time, maintaining a stable and level pelvis (A).

✳ Keep your shoulders away from your ears, and your head in line with your spine.

A

✳ Slightly tuck your tailbone under and squeeze your glutes, draw your abs in and lock your knees, pulling your kneecaps up your thighs.

DOUBLE LEG STRETCH

Benefits: strengthens your entire core, flattens your abs, and mobilises your shoulders and hips

- Lie on your back with your knees bent and hip-width apart.
- Exhale to bring one knee at a time up above your hips to the table-top position.
- Now exhale navel to spine, lift your head and shoulders off the floor, reaching your hands down towards your ankles (A).
- Inhale to prepare. Exhale and reach your arms back overhead while extending your legs, keeping your back on the floor (B).
- Inhale, bend your knees back to a table top, circling your arms back and around to reach towards your ankles (C) and (D).
- Continue in a flowing motion eight times.

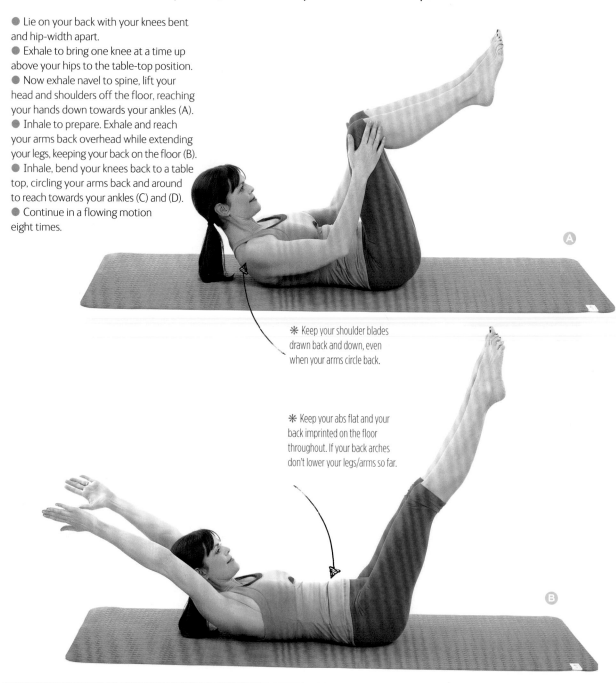

✳ Keep your shoulder blades drawn back and down, even when your arms circle back.

✳ Keep your abs flat and your back imprinted on the floor throughout. If your back arches don't lower your legs/arms so far.

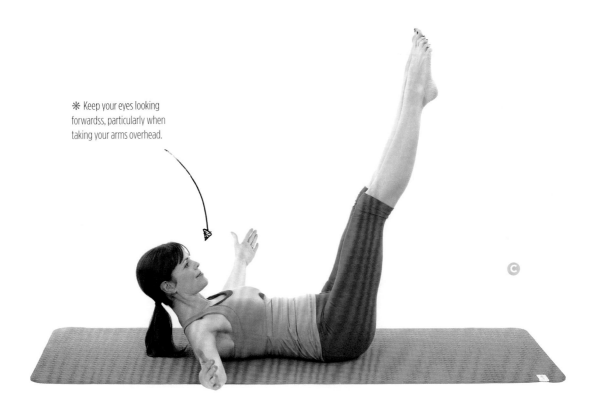

✳ Keep your eyes looking forwardss, particularly when taking your arms overhead.

C

BEGINNERS
● Start with your arms only, then your legs only, with your head up and hands by your sides. Gradually move on to the full exercise.

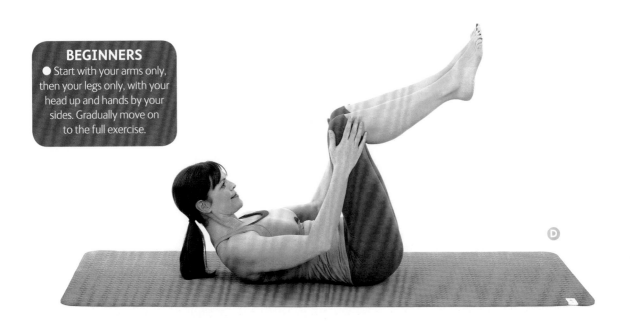

D

10-MINUTE ABS WORKOUT

Strengthen your abs, core and torso, tone your waist and
mobilise your spine, shoulders and hips with this abs workout

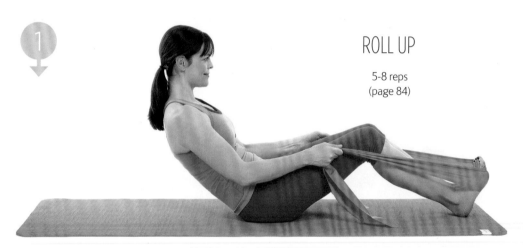

1

ROLL UP

5-8 reps
(page 84)

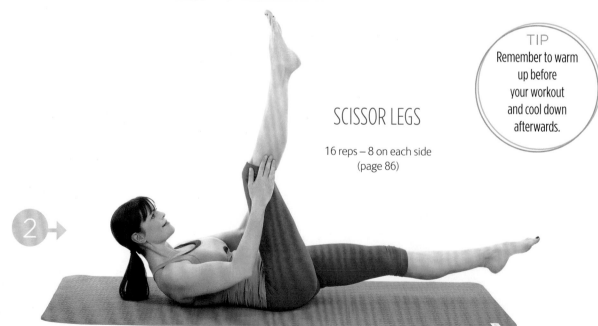

SCISSOR LEGS

16 reps – 8 on each side
(page 86)

2

TIP
Remember to warm
up before
your workout
and cool down
afterwards.

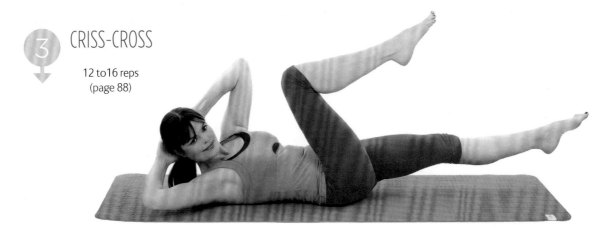

3 CRISS-CROSS

12 to16 reps
(page 88)

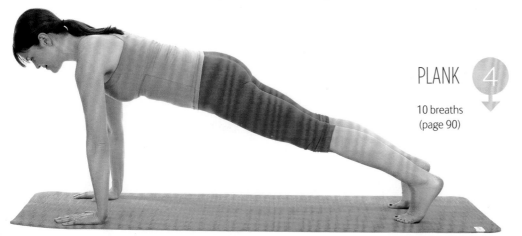

PLANK 4

10 breaths
(page 90)

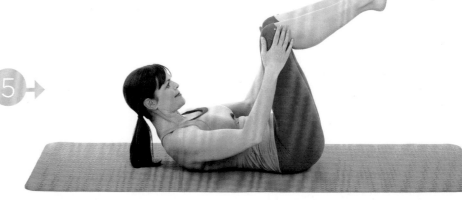

DOUBLE LEG STRETCH 5

8 reps
(page 92)

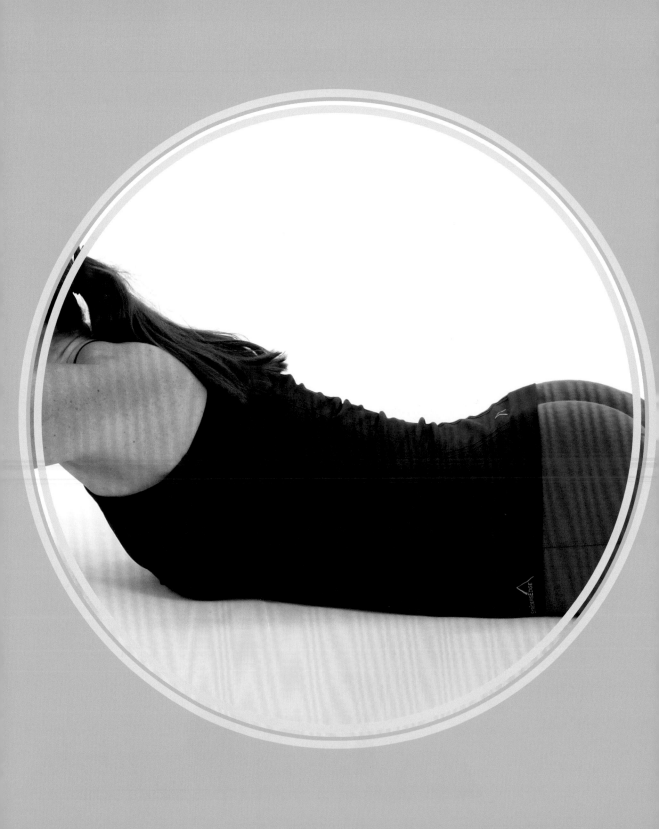

STRONG BACK

✳ A healthy back is supple and strong and Pilates improves both. Your spine is designed to move through flexion (bending forwards), extension (moving backwards) and rotation (moving sideways and twisting), but we tend to sit or stand with our spines in flexion (sofa slump!). As the spine moves, it draws fluid in and out of the vertebral discs, helping to keep them plump and healthy. Lack of movement does the opposite and can age your spine, making you stiff and prone to pain. When you practise Pilates, lengthen your spine, drawing your head away from your tailbone, decompressing your spine and aiding the movement of fluid.

These exercises work both the global muscles and local stabilising ones. If you have a back condition, practise the basic exercises for a few weeks to help build stability.

CAT STRETCH

Benefits: mobilises your entire spine

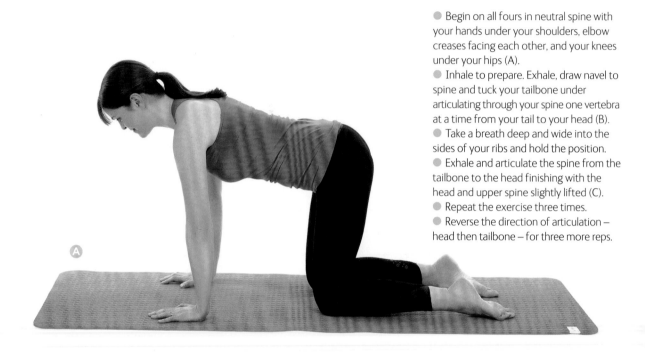

A

● Begin on all fours in neutral spine with your hands under your shoulders, elbow creases facing each other, and your knees under your hips (A).
● Inhale to prepare. Exhale, draw navel to spine and tuck your tailbone under articulating through your spine one vertebra at a time from your tail to your head (B).
● Take a breath deep and wide into the sides of your ribs and hold the position.
● Exhale and articulate the spine from the tailbone to the head finishing with the head and upper spine slightly lifted (C).
● Repeat the exercise three times.
● Reverse the direction of articulation – head then tailbone – for three more reps.

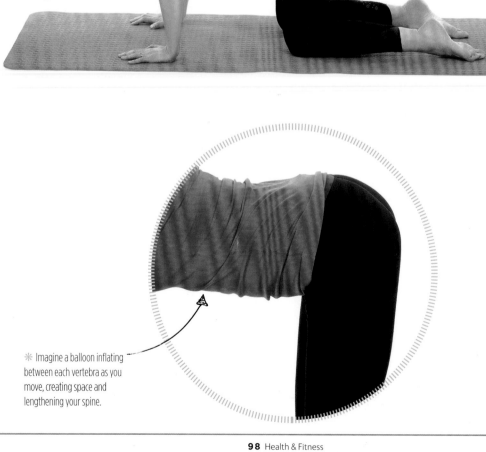

✳ Imagine a balloon inflating between each vertebra as you move, creating space and lengthening your spine.

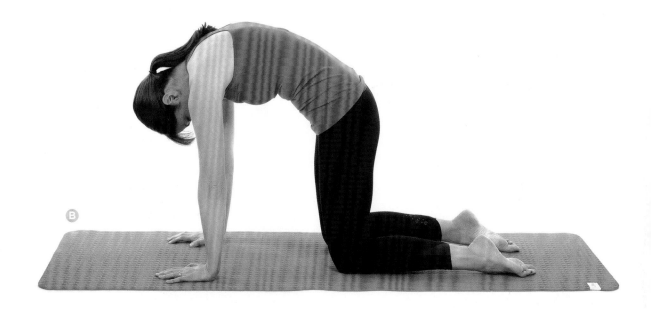

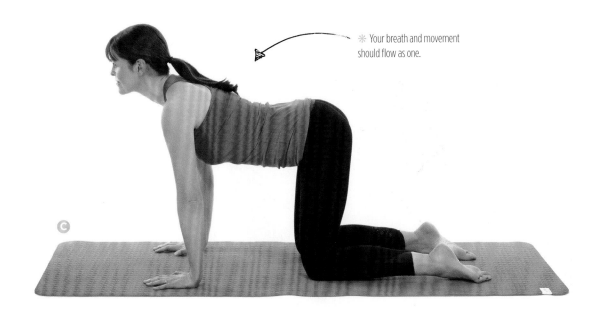

✳ Your breath and movement should flow as one.

BALANCE HOLD

Benefits: stabilises your pelvis and lumbar spine,
and strengthens your abs, shoulders and core

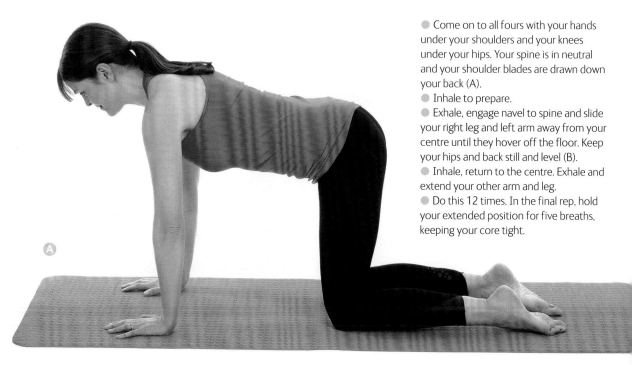

● Come on to all fours with your hands
under your shoulders and your knees
under your hips. Your spine is in neutral
and your shoulder blades are drawn down
your back (A).
● Inhale to prepare.
● Exhale, engage navel to spine and slide
your right leg and left arm away from your
centre until they hover off the floor. Keep
your hips and back still and level (B).
● Inhale, return to the centre. Exhale and
extend your other arm and leg.
● Do this 12 times. In the final rep, hold
your extended position for five breaths,
keeping your core tight.

Ⓐ

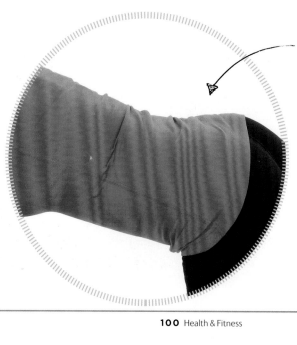

✳ Imagine you have four
glasses of water sitting on the
four corners of your spine – make
sure you don't spill a drop!

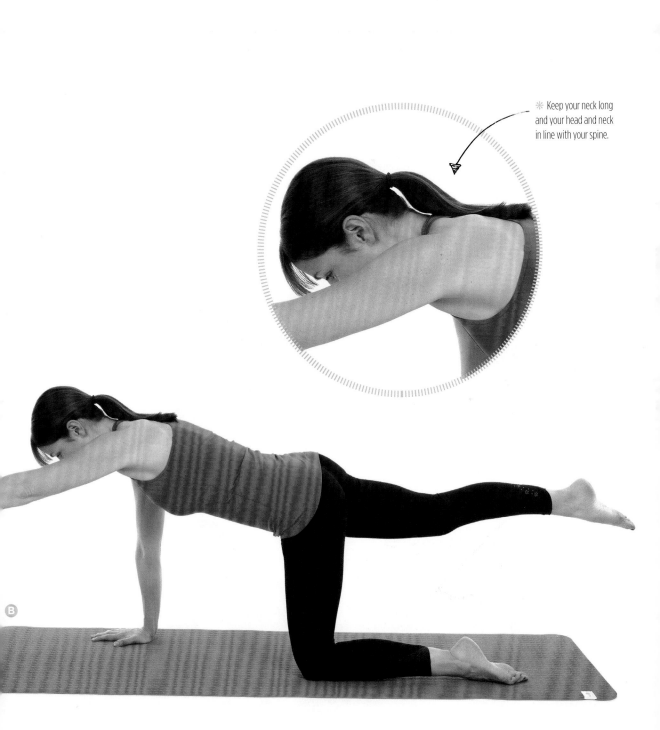

※ Keep your neck long and your head and neck in line with your spine.

B

BRIDGE

Benefits: mobilises your spine, strengthens your glutes and lengthens your hip flexors

● Lie on your back in neutral spine with your knees bent and feet and knees hip-width apart.
● Inhale to prepare.
● Exhale and draw navel to spine, tucking your tailbone to tilt your pelvis (A).
● Inhale back to neutral. Exhale and tilt as above, this time articulating a couple

of your vertebra off the floor (B).
● Inhale back.
● Exhale and roll one vertebra at a time off the floor until you make a straight line from your knee-to-hip-to-shoulder (C).
● Inhale to stay up and exhale to come back down one vertebra at a time.
● Repeat the exercise three to five times.

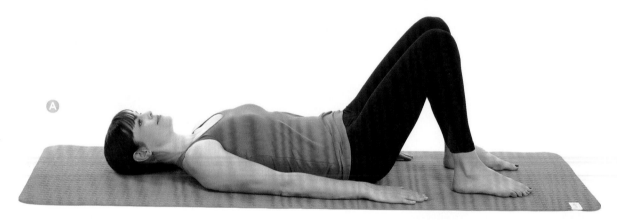

A

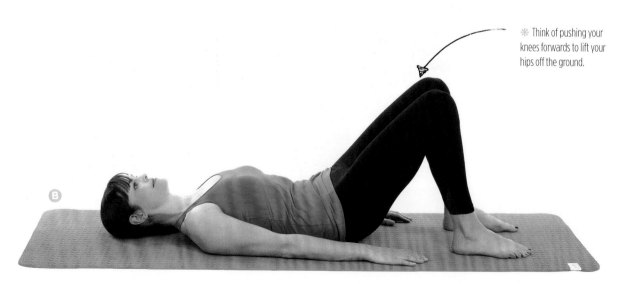

※ Think of pushing your knees forwards to lift your hips off the ground.

B

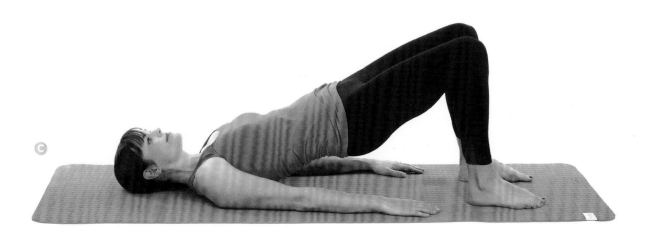

C

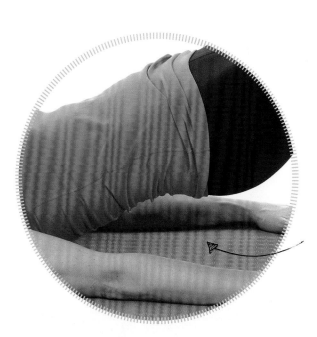

✳ Make sure you keep your tailbone tucked under as you're lifting and at the top. You should feel the effort in your glutes and hamstrings and not your back.

TOE TAPS THEN KNEES TO CHEST
Benefits: tones your abs and works your glutes

● Lie on your back in neutral with knees bent and hip-width apart.
● Exhale to lift one leg at a time into the table top position (A).
● Place your hands on your tummy with your thumbs on your bottom rib and your little fingers on your hips bones (inset).
● Inhale to prepare.
● Exhale and draw navel to spine, bringing your hips and ribs – thumb and little finger – closer together as you lower one foot to tap the floor (B).
● Inhale your leg back up and continue in time with your breath for six to eight reps on each side.

✳ Use your hands to feel that your abs stay tight and flattened. If your tummy muscles 'pop' up don't take your leg quite so low.

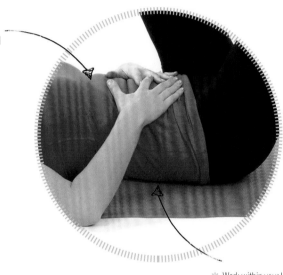

✳ Work within your limits. If you feel your back is about to arch bend your knee more, or don't take your leg quite so low.

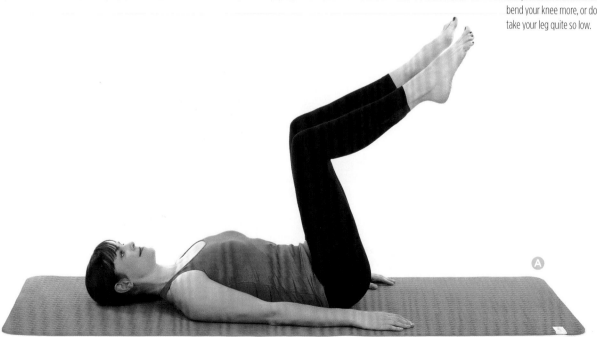

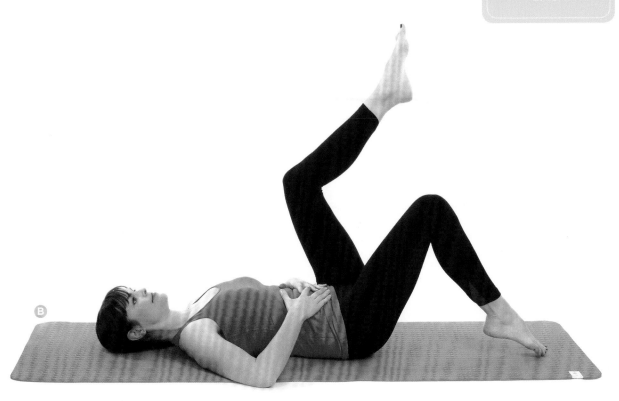

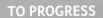

TO PROGRESS
● As with the main exercise, but straighten your leg as you lower it.

ALTERNATIVE
● Place your fingertips behind your ears and flex your head and shoulders forwards.
● Exhale to lower one foot towards the floor, inhale and return as in the main exercise.
● Keep your head and shoulders lifted for 12 to 16 reps.

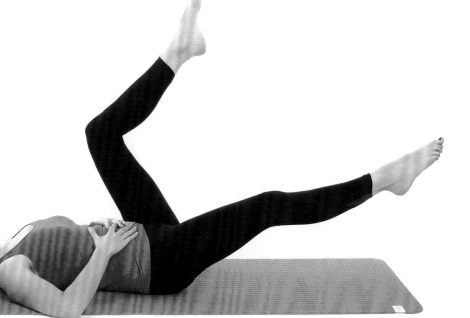

SWIMMING

Benefits: strengthens your core, particularly the muscles running up and down your spine. It also tones your glutes and mobilises your upper back

- Lie on your stomach with your legs hip-width apart with your toes pointed and slightly turned out. Think of turning out from the hip.
- Extend your arms overhead with your palms facing down (A).
- Inhale to prepare.
- Exhale and draw navel to spine – as if you're lifting your tummy button gently off the floor – as you reach your head, arms and both legs off the floor (B).
- Reach one arm and the opposite leg a little higher and then the other as if you're swimming, while inhaling for five kicks and exhaling for five kicks. This is one set (C).
- Repeat the exercise for five sets.

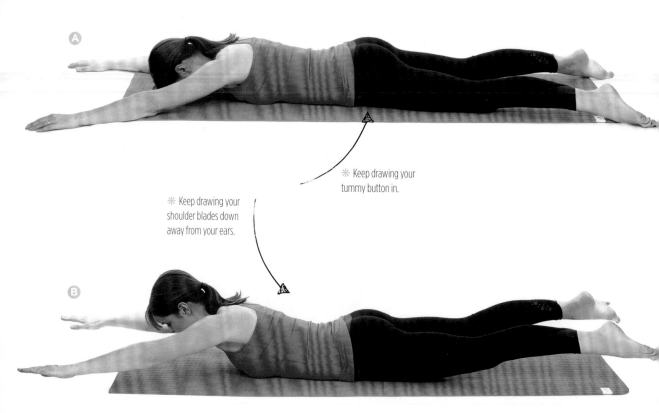

※ Keep drawing your tummy button in.

※ Keep drawing your shoulder blades down away from your ears.

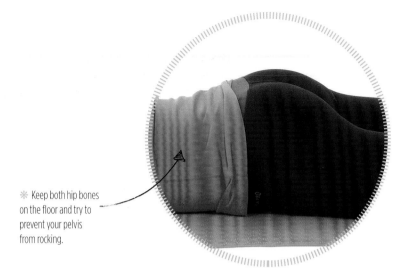

✳ Keep both hip bones on the floor and try to prevent your pelvis from rocking.

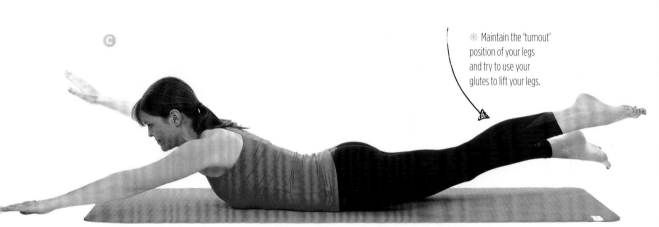

C

✳ Maintain the 'turnout' position of your legs and try to use your glutes to lift your legs.

BEGINNERS
● Begin in the start position as above, but keep one arm and the opposite leg on the floor as you exhale to lift the other, alternating the sides. Your head and neck should lift and lower in time with your arms. Repeat 10 on each side.

BREAST STROKE (WITH FLEX BAND)

Benefits: mobilises your upper back and shoulders,
and strengthens your spine and core muscles

- Lie on your stomach with your legs drawn together and your arms bent on the floor. Your finger tips should be approximately in line with your nose (A).
- Inhale to prepare.
- Exhale and gently draw navel to spine as you push your hands into the floor and draw your shoulder blades down, away from your ears, extending your head and shoulders off the floor (B).
- Inhale and lower your back to the start.
- Repeat the exercise eight times.

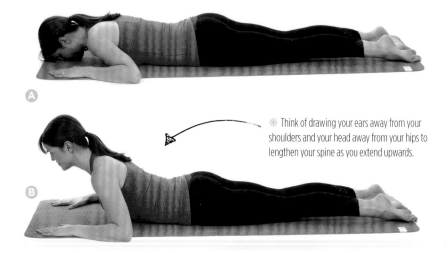

✳ Think of drawing your ears away from your shoulders and your head away from your hips to lengthen your spine as you extend upwards.

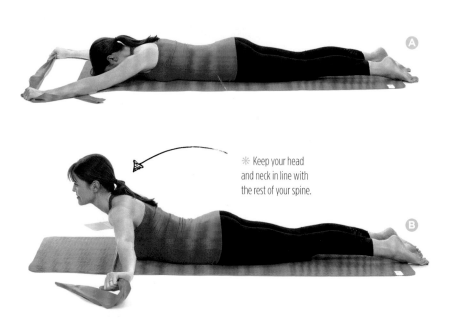

✳ Keep your head and neck in line with the rest of your spine.

TO PROGRESS

- Lie on your stomach with your legs drawn together and your arms overhead, holding the ends of the band (A).
- Inhale to prepare.
- Exhale, draw navel to spine as if pulling your tummy button off the floor. Lengthen and lift your shoulders off the floor while pulling the band out to the sides until it touches your chest (B).
- Inhale to stay up.
- Exhale back to the start position.
- Repeat five to eight times.

SHELL STRETCH

Benefits: decompresses your spine, relaxes and
stretches muscles on the back of your body

From the breast stroke, lying on your
tummy, place your hands under your
shoulders and draw navel to spine as
you press your bottom back on to your
heels, your head on to the mat. Start
with your arms reaching forward for
a few breaths (A).

Then take your fingertips down to
your toes and let your shoulders relax
completely (B).

Take up to 10 deep, slow breaths
allowing your body to relax.

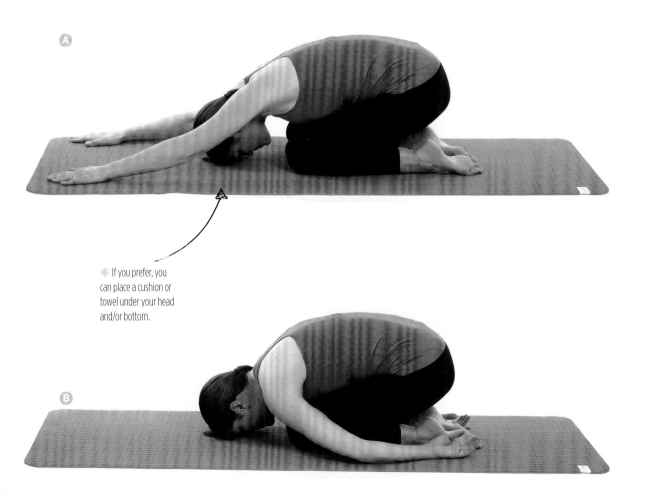

✳ If you prefer, you
can place a cushion or
towel under your head
and/or bottom.

10-MINUTE BACK WORKOUT

Mobilise your upper back, stabilise your pelvis and lumbar spine,
and strengthen your core muscles with this back workout

TIP
Remember to warm
up before
your workout
and cool down
afterwards.

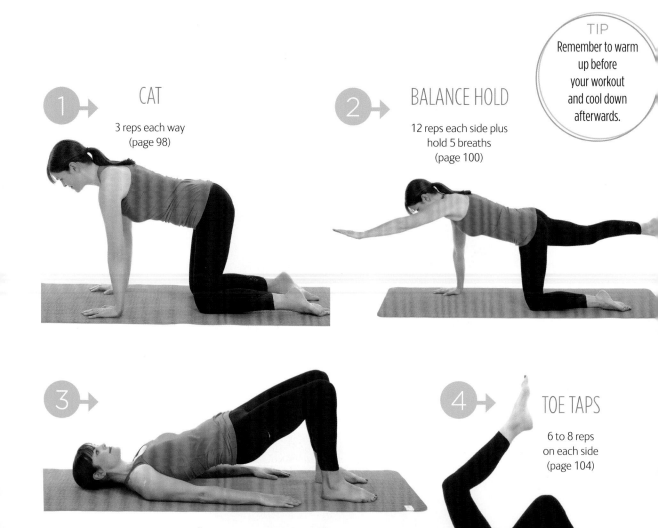

1 **CAT**

3 reps each way
(page 98)

2 **BALANCE HOLD**

12 reps each side plus
hold 5 breaths
(page 100)

3

BRIDGE

3 to 5 reps
(page 102)

4 **TOE TAPS**

6 to 8 reps
on each side
(page 104)

SWIMMING

8 reps
(page 106)

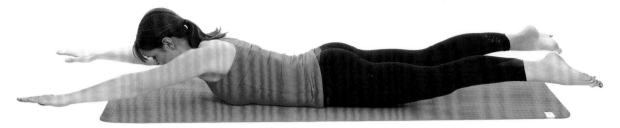

BREAST STROKE

8 reps
(page 108)

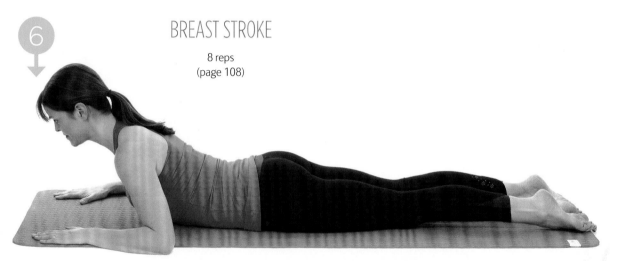

SHELL STRETCH

10 breaths
(page 109)

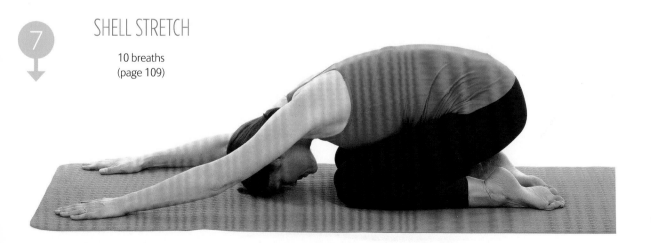

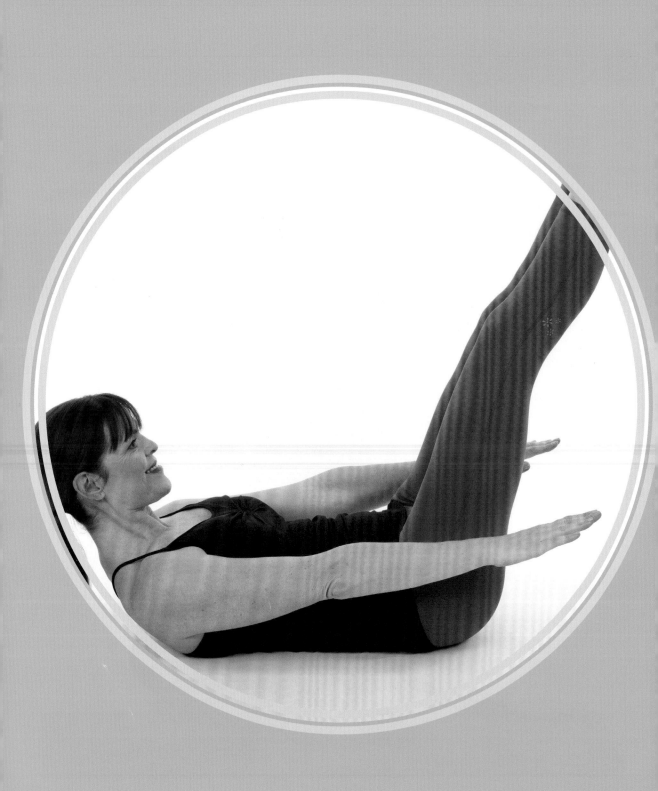

TOTAL BODY

✳ This chapter is designed to work as many muscles and joints as possible in 10 minutes! Classic exercises, such as the 'Roll down to push up' (page 114) and '100' (page 118) are both unchanged from Pilates' original exercises and are challenging and effective. Always work within your limits using any progressions offered. Build up gradually and with control – remember your Pilates principles!

If time allows, you could repeat the circuit (page 124) twice and add in extra push-ups to the 'Roll down to push up' exercise (page 114), building up to three to four sets of 10 push-ups. Or you could tag on an extra workout from one of the other chapters of this book to really zone in on one part of your body.

INSIDE...

Roll down to push up

Side bend

100

Lunge & biceps

Double leg lift

10-minute workout

ROLL DOWN TO PUSH UP

Benefits: mobilises your spine, stretches the entire back of your body, and strengthens your shoulders, arms and core

- Stand with your feet and knees hip-width apart (A).
- Inhale to prepare.
- Exhale to roll down one vertebra at a time until your hands are by your toes or shins according to your flexibility (B).
- Inhale to walk your hands out to plank position in three hand 'steps' (C).

✳ Keep your weight in the centre of your feet as you roll down and your abs drawn in.

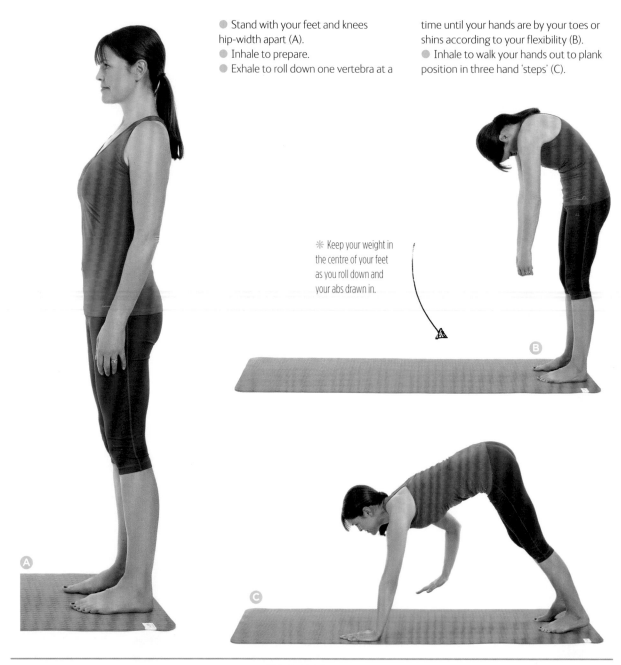

✳ For the push-up, make sure you keep your abs drawn in, your shoulders away from your ears and your spine in neutral. Exhale as you push up and imagine you're blowing yourself off the floor.

✳ Keep your knees 'soft' and bend them a little more if you have any tightness in your back.

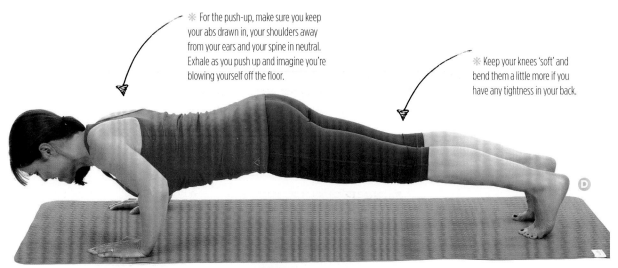

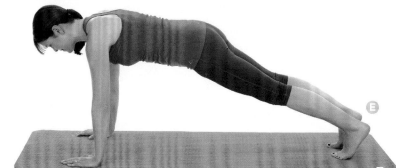

● In full press-up position, inhale and lower your chest between your hands (D).
● Exhale navel to spine, push up and repeat three times (E).
● Now reverse the steps to roll back up one vertebra at a time to standing using your abdominal muscles to rebuild your spine.
● Repeat the entire process three times.

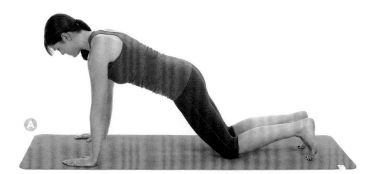

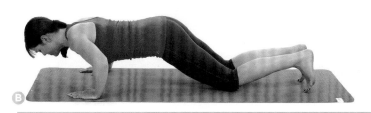

BEGINNER VERSION
● Follow the steps opposite to come down on to the mat.
● Lower your knees to the floor, keeping them behind your hips and your spine in neutral (A).
● Inhale to lower your chest between your hands (B).
● Exhale to push back up and repeat three times before coming back to standing, as opposite.

SIDE BEND

Benefits: strengthens and tightens your core, particularly the oblique muscles of your waist. It also strengthens the muscles of your shoulders, inner thighs and hips

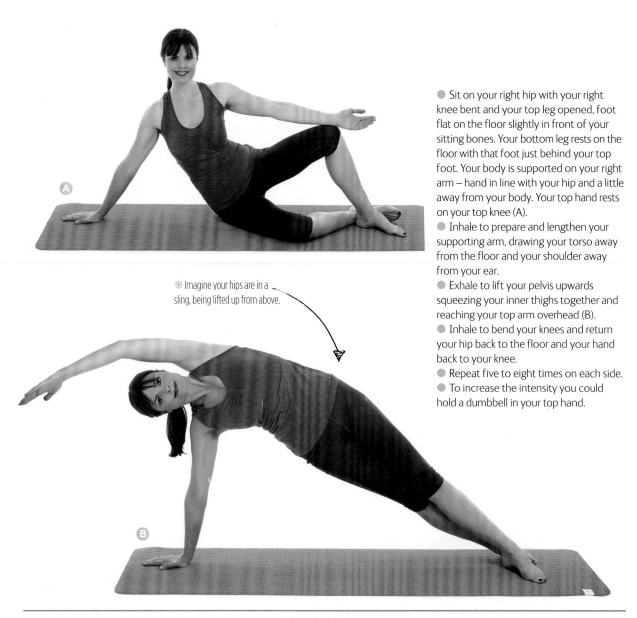

● Sit on your right hip with your right knee bent and your top leg opened, foot flat on the floor slightly in front of your sitting bones. Your bottom leg rests on the floor with that foot just behind your top foot. Your body is supported on your right arm – hand in line with your hip and a little away from your body. Your top hand rests on your top knee (A).

● Inhale to prepare and lengthen your supporting arm, drawing your torso away from the floor and your shoulder away from your ear.

● Exhale to lift your pelvis upwards squeezing your inner thighs together and reaching your top arm overhead (B).

● Inhale to bend your knees and return your hip back to the floor and your hand back to your knee.

● Repeat five to eight times on each side.

● To increase the intensity you could hold a dumbbell in your top hand.

✳ Imagine your hips are in a sling, being lifted up from above.

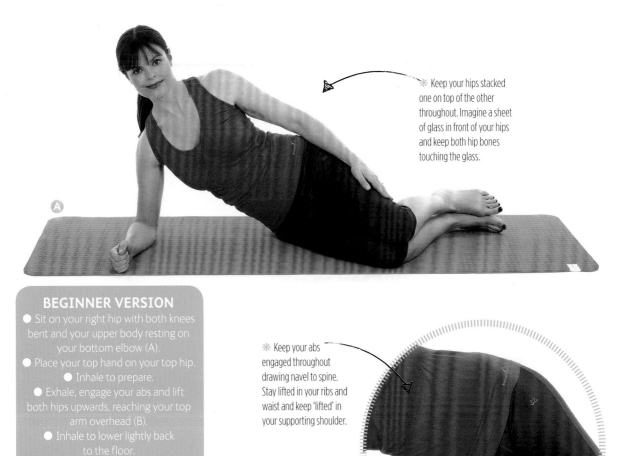

✳ Keep your hips stacked one on top of the other throughout. Imagine a sheet of glass in front of your hips and keep both hip bones touching the glass.

A

BEGINNER VERSION

- Sit on your right hip with both knees bent and your upper body resting on your bottom elbow (A).
- Place your top hand on your top hip.
- Inhale to prepare.
- Exhale, engage your abs and lift both hips upwards, reaching your top arm overhead (B).
- Inhale to lower lightly back to the floor.
- Repeat five to eight times on each side.

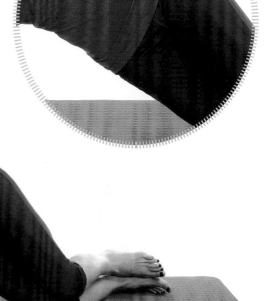

✳ Keep your abs engaged throughout drawing navel to spine. Stay lifted in your ribs and waist and keep 'lifted' in your supporting shoulder.

B

100

Benefits: it's perhaps the best known Pilates exercise which strengthens your entire core and flattens your abs

- Lie on your back with your knees bent and feet and knees hip-width apart.
- Exhale to contract your abs and bring both knees up to a table top (A).
- Now exhale to lift your head, shoulders and arms off the floor.
- Begin to beat your arms as if pressing up and down on heavy springs (B).
- Inhale for five arm beats and exhale for five arm beats building up to 100 beats.
- Beginners should start with 50 beats building up to 100.

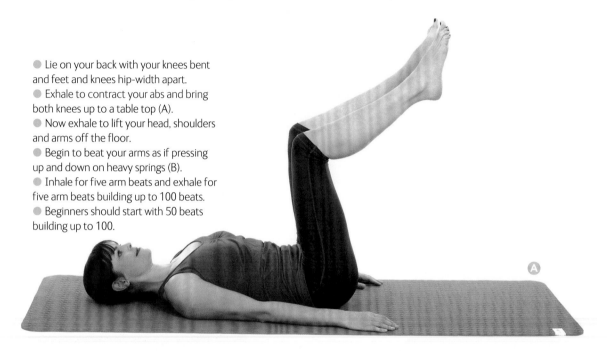

A

✳ Keep navel to spine throughout and your shoulders away from your ears, shoulder blades drawn down.

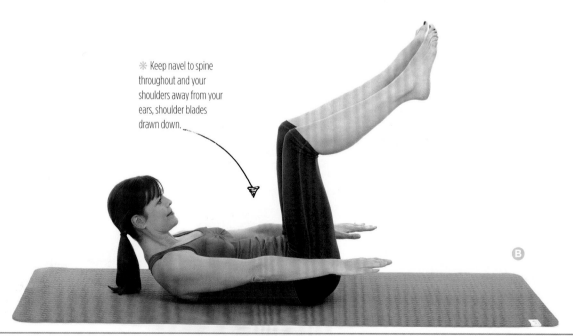

B

TO PROGRESS

● Straighten your legs out while keeping your abs flat and your back imprinted on the floor.
● Keep your abs contracted throughout and your legs strong – knees locked and legs lengthened away from your body.
● To progress further lower your straightened legs towards the floor as far as you can without tensing your back.

✳ Breathe into the sides of your ribs, inhaling through your nose and exhaling through your lips.

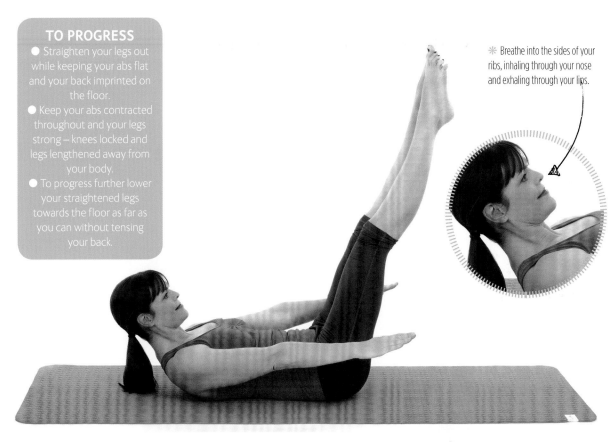

ADD A BAND

◉ Place a flex band flat across your shins holding on to the ends with your thumb and forefinger.
◉ As you beat your arms for the 100 count, gently pull against band.
◉ This version is challenging for the abs so be sure to keep your spine imprinted on the floor and your abs flat.

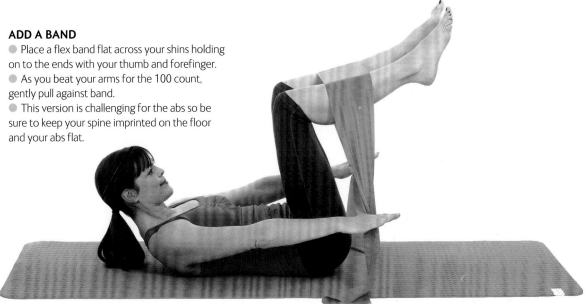

LUNGE & BICEPS

Benefits: strengthens and tightens your bottom, thighs, front of arms and shoulders

● Stand with a flex band under your right foot, holding an end in each hand with your palms facing each other (A).
● As you exhale and engage your core, step back with your left foot, bending both knees to an approximate right angle. At the same time bend your elbows, bringing your fists to your shoulders (B).
● Inhale as you step back to the start position.
● Repeat the exercise 10 to 12 times on each leg.

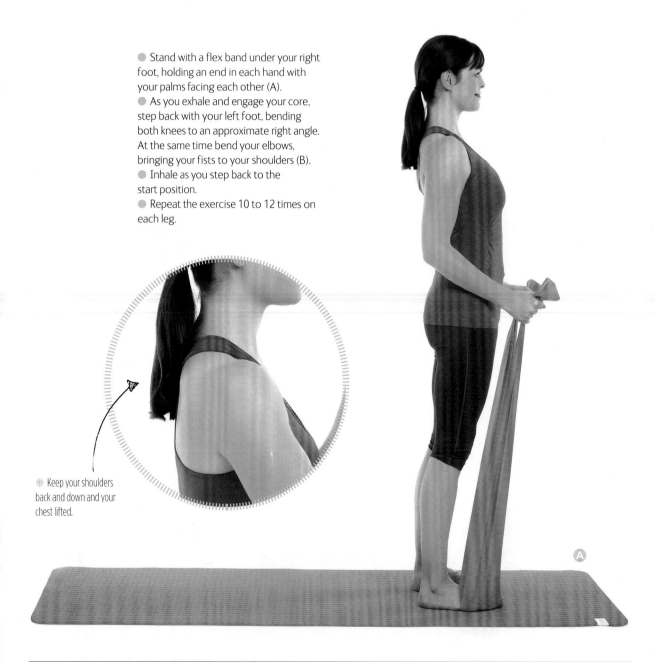

✳ Keep your shoulders back and down and your chest lifted.

Ⓐ

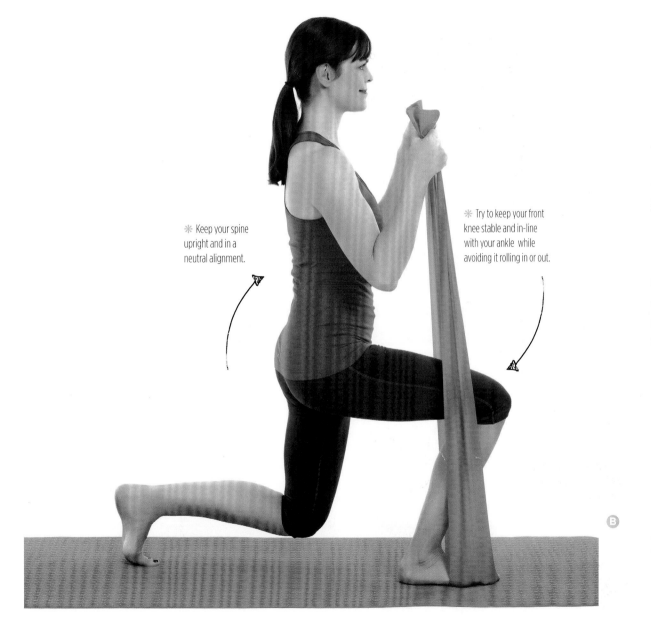

✳ Keep your spine upright and in a neutral alignment.

✳ Try to keep your front knee stable and in-line with your ankle while avoiding it rolling in or out.

Ⓑ

DOUBLE LEG LIFT

Benefits: strengthens your core, particularly the
obliques (waist), and tones your legs and inner thighs

● Lie on your side with your head on an outstretched arm, with your legs together and your toes just in front of your hips. Your top hand is on the floor in front of your chest and your underneath hand has its palm facing upwards (A).
● Inhale to prepare.
● Exhale, engage navel to spine and squeeze your legs together as you lift

them both from the floor (B).
● Inhale and gently lower your legs back to the floor.
● Continue in time with your breath eight times.
● Now hold your legs in the 'up' position and lift and lower the top leg eight times (C).
● If you want more resistance use a flex band.

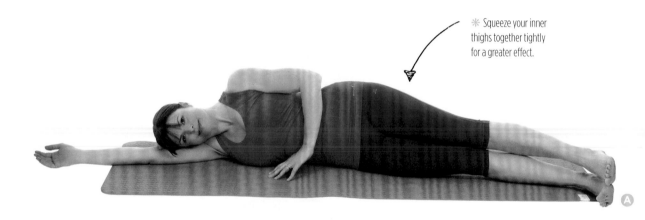

✳ Squeeze your inner
thighs together tightly
for a greater effect.

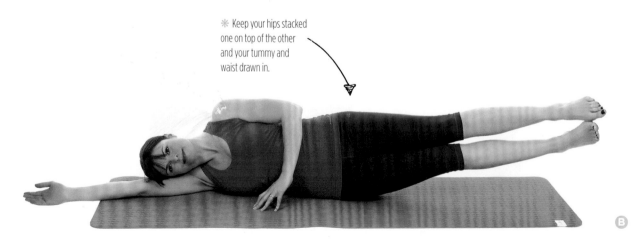

✳ Keep your hips stacked
one on top of the other
and your tummy and
waist drawn in.

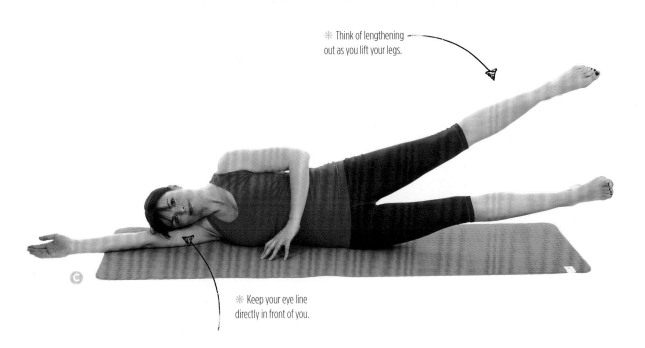

✳ Think of lengthening out as you lift your legs.

✳ Keep your eye line directly in front of you.

TO PROGRESS
● Do the exercises as above but with your top arm resting along your side.

10-MINUTE TOTAL BODY WORKOUT

Strengthen, trim and tone your whole body with this intense workout

TIP
Remember to warm up before your workout and cool down afterwards.

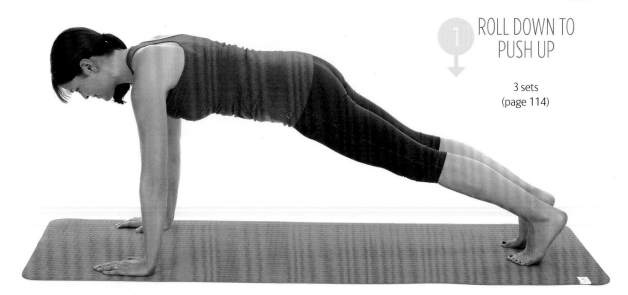

1 ROLL DOWN TO PUSH UP

3 sets
(page 114)

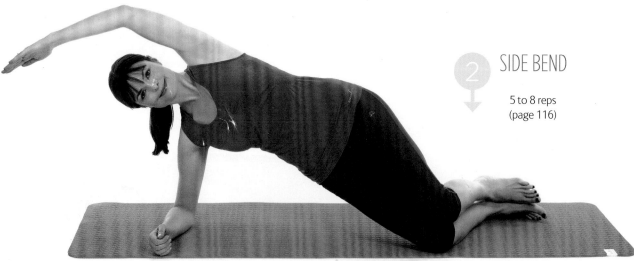

2 SIDE BEND

5 to 8 reps
(page 116)

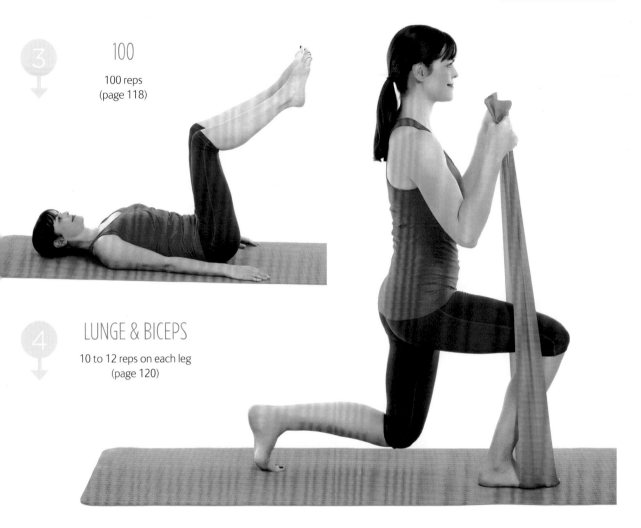

3   100

100 reps
(page 118)

4   LUNGE & BICEPS

10 to 12 reps on each leg
(page 120)

5   DOUBLE LEG LIFT

8 reps then 8 reps
(page 122)

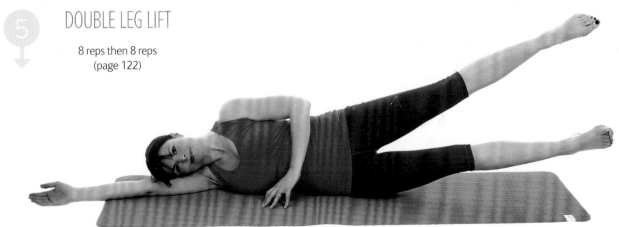

STRETCH OUT

It's the part of our workouts that we often skip. But taking time to stretch will restore your muscles and prevent any injuries

1 HAMSTRINGS

● Lie on your back and wrap a flex band around your right foot.
● Straighten your right leg up towards the ceiling until you feel a stretch down the back of your thigh, gently pulling on the band to increase the stretch (A).
● Hold for several deep breaths and then swap sides.

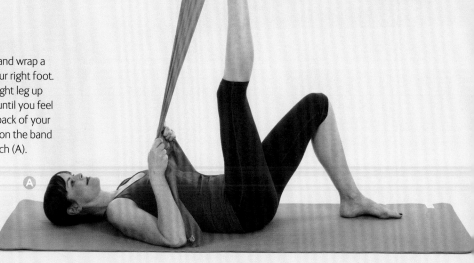

2 GLUTE STRETCH

● Stay on your back and cross your left ankle over your bent right knee.
● Draw both knees in towards your chest then link your hands together around the back of your right thigh (A).
● Hold and take several deep breaths then change legs.

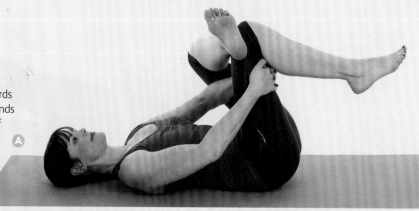

3 SIDE TWIST

● Lie on your back with your arms extended out at shoulder height and your knees bent.
● Slowly lower your legs over to the left, allowing your right foot to lift off the floor, and turn your head to the right (A).
● Hold for several breaths on each side and repeat the exercise two to three times.

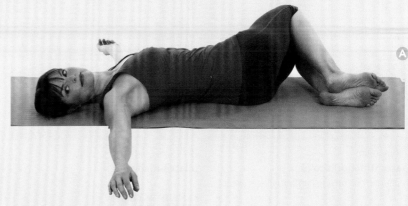

4 HIP FLEXOR RELEASE

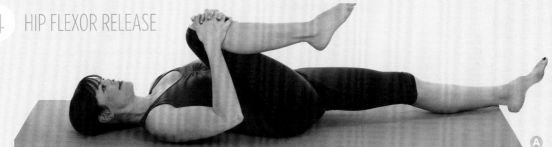

● Lying on your back, draw your right knee into your chest and hold on to it with your hands.
● Lengthen your left leg out on the floor (A).
● Take three deep breaths, squeezing your right knee to your chest as you exhale and completely relaxing your left leg. This is a passive stretch for this leg.
● Repeat the exercise on the other side.

5 CHEST RELEASE

● Take a cushion, rolled up towel or soft ball and place it under your upper back, around shoulder blade level (A).
● Lie back over the padding allowing your chest to lift and your shoulders to open (B).
● Stretch your legs out long and relax (C).
● Stay for as long as possible and take deep breaths feeling your chest expand and your shoulders open.

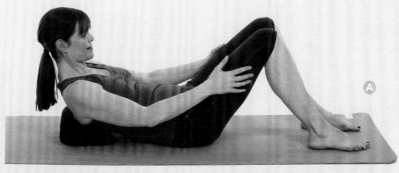

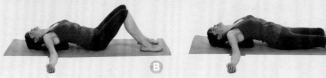

Directory

APPAREL

● Asquith
asquithlondon.co.uk
Organic cotton and bamboo Pilates wear

● Boobydoo
boobydoo.co.uk
Online sports bra store

● Casall
casall.co.uk
High-quality Swedish fitness wear

● Lululemon
lululemon.co.uk
Yoga-inspired fitness wear

● Shock Absorber
shockabsorber.co.uk
Fitness sports bras

● Striders Edge
stridersedge.co.uk
Pilates, yoga and outdoor wear

● Sweaty Betty
sweatybetty.co.uk
Online fitness wear boutique

● USA Pro
sportsdirect.com
Affordable home fitness wear

● Wellicious
welicious.com
Luxury Pilates, yoga and loungewear

● Lovestretch
lovestretch.co.uk
The latest stretch collections

PILATES EQUIPMENT

● Pilates Mad
pilates-mad.com

● Physical Company
physicalcompany.co.uk

PILATES ORGANISATIONS

● Pilates Near You
pilatesnearyou.co.uk
Find a local Pilates class to suit your goals

● Pilates Foundation
pilatesfoundation.com
Education and teacher training

● Pilates Institute
pilates-institute.hu
Classes and teacher training

● Body Control Pilates
bodycontrolpilates.com
Classes, teacher training,
healthy back classes

FOOD AND SUPPLMENTS

● Reflex nutrition
reflex-nutrition.com
Quality sports supplements

● Udo's Choice Ultimate Oil Blend
udoschoice.co.uk
Blend of omega 3, 6, 9 essential fatty acids

● Vitabiotics
vitabiotics.com
Vitamin supplements for women

● Vita Coco
vitacoco.com/uk
Rehydrating coconut water drink

● Heath & Heather
healthandheather.co.uk
Award-winning herbal teas

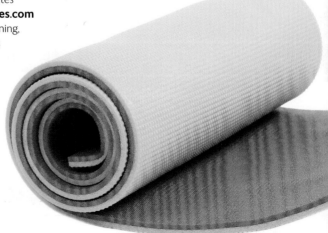

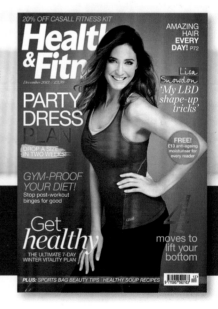

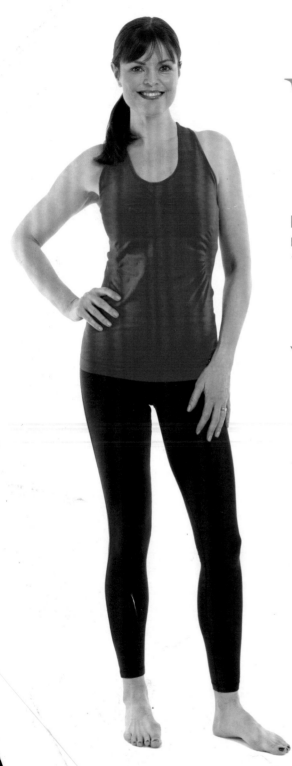

Well done

We hope that you've enjoyed exercising with the Pilates system and are already feeling its benefits. Remember, 10 minutes is better than no minutes, so keep this book handy to make the most of any unexpected windows of opportunity. We recommend you try to do at least one 10-minute Pilates workout, five days a week.

You could do the Total Body workout to help you relax after a busy day at work. You could tag the Flat Abs workout on after a run, or do the Amazing Arms workout to energise you at lunch time. However you choose to use this book, we hope you'll continue to discover the amazing benefits of Pilates for a happier, healthier and more balanced body for life.

✳

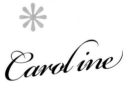